THE
HEALTH
DEBATE

Second edition

THE
HEALTH
DEBATE

Second edition

David J. Hunter

First edition published in 2008

Second edition published in Great Britain in 2016 by

Policy Press
University of Bristol
1-9 Old Park Hill
Bristol BS2 8BB
UK
t: +44 (0)117 954 5940
e: pp-info@bristol.ac.uk
www.policypress.co.uk

North American office:
Policy Press
c/o The University of Chicago Press
1427 East 60th Street
Chicago, IL 60637, USA
t: +1 773 702 7700
f: +1 773-702-9756
e:sales@press.uchicago.edu
www.press.uchicago.edu

British Library Cataloguing in Publication Data
A catalogue record for this book is available from the British Library.

Library of Congress Cataloging-in-Publication Data
A catalog record for this book has been requested.

ISBN 978-1-4473-2697-7 paperback
ISBN 978-1-4473-2700-4 ePub
ISBN 978-1-4473-2699-1 Mobi

Cover design by Policy Press
Front cover: istock
Printed and bound in Great Britain by CMP, Poole
Policy Press uses environmentally responsible print partners

For Jacqui, Eve and Miles and my colleagues in the
Centre for Public Policy and Health, Durham University,
without whose encouragement, support, understanding
and forbearance the book would not
have been completed.

Medicine is a social science, and politics nothing else but medicine on a large scale.

Rudolf Virchow
(1821–1902)

Contents

List of boxes

About the author

David Hunter is Professor of Health Policy and Management at Durham University where he is Director of the Centre for Public Policy and Health located in the School of Medicine, Pharmacy and Health. He is a Wolfson Fellow in the Wolfson Research Institute for Health and Wellbeing, and Senior Fellow of the Durham Global Policy Institute. He is Deputy Director of Fuse, the UKCRC (Clinical Research Collaboration) Centre for Translational Research in Public Health. David's research interests include partnership working in the NHS, the impact of Health and Wellbeing Boards, prioritisation in public health spending in local government, health system reform, transformational change in the NHS, and commissioning in primary care and in public health.

David is a special advisor to WHO Europe and in 2014 his Centre at Durham was designated a WHO Collaborating Centre in Complex Health Systems Research, Knowledge and Action. Since 2008 David has been a Non Executive Director of the National Institute for Health and Care Excellence (NICE), and since 2009 he has been an Appointed Governor on the Council of Governors, South Tees Hospitals NHS Foundation Trust. He is an Honorary Member of the Faculty of Public Health and a Fellow of the Royal College of Physicians in Edinburgh.

Acknowledgements

There are many people stretching back over many years to whom I owe a great debt both in the production of the first edition of this book and now its second edition. There are too many to thank individually and it would be invidious to single out a few for special mention. But I make an exception for two people to whom I owe a special debt of gratitude in shaping my thinking and career. My late father, Drummond Hunter (1918–2002), who worked as a hospital administrator, as they were then called, in the Scottish NHS and subsequently as a civil servant in the Scottish Home and Health Department at the Scottish Office, not only introduced me to the fascinations of the NHS as a complex system but also demonstrated the value and importance of being a passionate yet critical friend of the NHS. He was truly a reflective practitioner without parallel especially at a time of significant, and often controversial, change in the NHS during the 1970s and 1980s.

The other person to whom I owe much gratitude is the late Raymond Illsley (1920–2013). Raymond was the external examiner for my PhD thesis which examined the workings of the Scottish NHS following its first reorganisation in 1974. He subsequently proved instrumental in giving me my first academic job at the University of Aberdeen where he was Professor of Sociology and Director of the MRC Medical Sociology Unit which was a training ground for many talented medical sociologists who went on to acquire national and international reputations. Raymond's 1980 Rock Carling Lecture, 'Professional or public health? Sociology in health and medicine', remains, in my view, as relevant and insightful now as it was then. Unusually for a medical sociologist, he saw the importance of studying the policy process, organisation and management structures, and recognised the difficulties in doing so. Both his, and my father's, spirit have been to the fore in writing this book – as much in evidence in the second edition as the first which is surely testimony to their lasting influence and inspiration.

Finally, turning to the present, I want to thank my colleagues at Durham University for their continuing support, encouragement and friendship over the many years I have been there. It has proved a fertile setting to observe the rapidly changing NHS and I feel privileged to have been in a position which has allowed me to do so with considerable freedom. Last, but not least, I thank my PA, Gill McGowan, who provided invaluable administrative support in producing this second edition and ensured that I kept time free wherever possible in a busy schedule to work on the book. I leave it to others to judge whether the effort has been worthwhile. Of course, I take full responsibility for any gaps, weaknesses or errors that may remain.

David J. Hunter
October 2015

Foreword

Very many people have become bewildered by the pace of change of the National Health Service and increasingly doubt whether the changes they are having to get used to will have any positive benefit for them. Of course, the world in which health care is delivered today is a very different world to that in which the NHS was set up by Aneurin Bevan, and change is necessary. The system cannot just stand still. But in responding to change there is a need for policy makers not to forget the collective action ideal that David Hunter quotes as inspiring the work of Bevan and his contemporaries.

What has been lacking in recent health policy making has been any effort to engineer change in a slow and systematic way, and to evaluate what has occurred. It is naïve to argue that politicians should leave the health service alone. What use is politics if it does not involve a quest to improve public policies? And health policies are among the most important public policies for us all. Moreover, as the long debate about how the health service is controlled has shown, political abdication implies the acceptance of professional dominance. Professionals have interests and do not always 'know best'. Here lie then many of the contradictions and dilemmas with which this book is concerned.

This second edition of the book is necessary because the pace of change in health policy has not slowed since the first edition. The end, in 2010, of the period of Labour Party dominance was succeeded by more policy change. The Conservative–Liberal Democrat coalition came into power with no obvious alternative agenda, but then proceeded to produce the controversial Health and Social Care Act (2012). As David Hunter shows, this legislation combined a commitment to advance further the process of private health provision, by no means absent in Labour policy making, with another phase of structural reform. Amendments following controversy over the initial Bill further complicated the process, leaving confusion in its wake. In the 2015 election, the Conservatives acquired power, without the need for a coalition ally. While they came in with no new agenda for the health service, they made clear their continuing commitment to both austerity and the private provision of public services. We are now in a period of uncertainty, in which an additional dimension has been introduced by developments in respect of devolution to Scotland, and to a lesser extent, Wales. Promises are also being made, which the book addresses with a cautious scepticism (that I share), about some delegation to local government. Diversity seems desirable, but, as the book shows, it tends to prompt political concerns about the so-called 'postcode lottery'. Turbulence is likely to continue for the National Health Service.

David Hunter is a scholar whose work has long involved an appreciation of the problems that have been rooted in too strong a professional dominance within health services. But he convincingly questions the alternative dominance of classical economics-based thinking about how to develop rational policy, nowadays reinforced by the intrusion of the simplistic economism of public choice theory into how many people analyse political and administrative behaviour. In any case, he suggests that many ideas from this direction have been taken up with little systematic thinking, let alone effective testing of their impact. In practice, hyperactive politics, not rational decision making, has driven the system. Market models, or indeed rampant commercialism, without consideration of whether these deliver the 'choice' they are believed to promise, have dominated so-called 'reform'. This book rightly questions whether choice (an ideal accepted by all but the most paternalistic providers) necessarily implies a need for competition, let alone competition in which private (for-profit) providers are a necessary part. The latter have become – surprise, surprise – the most vociferous advocates of health policy change. Meanwhile, others (such as academic economists who – we hope – do not stand to gain from privatisation) have subscribed to the mantra that it does not matter who provides services so long as the health service remains tax funded. A very important aspect of this book is that it shows the dangers for the public service ideal that lurk in that point of view.

As David Hunter points out, international comparative surveys tend to score the British health service high, and the American health system (the source of much of the privatisation pressure) very low. While that should not engender British complacency, it does point to the importance of preserving the essence of the original National Health Service. Here is a book that provides evidence for that perspective.

Michael Hill
Series Editor

ONE

Key challenges facing health systems

Introduction

The reader may wonder why another book on health policy is deemed necessary given the numerous texts already available, many of them updated versions of earlier ones. It is a fair question, particularly when this text is a second edition and falls into that category. In its defence, it attempts to do a different job. The aim of the book is to explore four key contemporary debates evident in health systems and consider how they have shaped the way in which such systems have evolved over time and continue to evolve. It is not a traditional comparative text since its principal focus is on health policy developments in the UK, with selective use made of examples from other countries and health systems where appropriate and of particular illustrative value. Most of the examples from outside the UK are drawn from other European health systems as well as from arrangements in North America, Australia and New Zealand.

The British NHS celebrated its 67th birthday in July 2015, but this book is not a history of its development or achievements over this period. Many existing texts already admirably serve this purpose, notably Baggott (2004), Ham (2004) and Klein (2006), and there is little to be gained by going over much the same ground, although there is some inevitable overlap. However, what sets the present book apart is a focus on a number of what might be termed policy cleavages that are evident in health and health care policy and in the development of health systems, and which are the subject of lengthy, often acrimonious and inconclusive, debate. The book is structured around four of these cleavages. They are:

- the balance between health care and health, whereby the latter is invariably overshadowed by the former in terms of political and media attention, professional lobbying, resource flows and public concern;
- the funding and organisation of health care systems and the mix of public and private arrangements, and the ever-changing balance between these;
- the ways in which health systems prioritise or ration health care and the degree to which this is undertaken explicitly or implicitly;
- the growing commodification of health as a market-style consumer good in which notions of choice and competition compete with, and may even be replacing, notions of collectivism and solidarity.

Running through each of these cleavages or debates is a tension between the public realm and private realm that gets played out in discourses on the role and limits of government on the one hand, and on the role of individuals in taking responsibility for their health and in exercising choice on the other. This tension is illustrated in the following example. How far, for instance, should the notion of stewardship apply to health systems where, according to the World Health Organisation (WHO), the key role of any government is the protection of the health of its population? Many policy makers take the view that this is a perfectly legitimate role for government and that it constitutes the hallmark of good government in a civilised society (Nuffield Council on Bioethics 2007). Others, however, reject this view in favour of one that states that governments have no business in health (or indeed any other domain with the exception perhaps of national security) and that it should be left to markets and individuals making personal choices to achieve optimal decisions. This is the neoliberal view that has been in the ascendant in many countries over the past 25 years or so.

Health systems the world over continue to attract attention from policy makers anxious to contain their costs at the same time as improving their efficiency, raising their quality and becoming more responsive to patient and public preferences. And all this at a time when expectations of what modern health care can do for people continue to rise. The common pressures of modern medicine centre on the financial and ethical choices of how limited resources ought to be distributed, and how a better balance can be found between treating ill-health on the one hand and promoting health on the other. These pressures are resulting in different countries moving to broadly common solutions. Of course, the solutions then need to be tailored to particular socioeconomic and political circumstances, values, cultures and historical traditions.

Reformers have never been more keen, if not desperate, to find solutions to a series of seemingly intractable and complex problems besetting health systems. Indeed, their insatiable appetite for solutions has fuelled a global industry of consultants whose fortunes are made by devising, and then furiously selling, the latest 'must-have' management fad or fashion.

Defining a health system

In its use of the term 'health system', this book views health in a broad sense and eschews a narrow conception of health care. Health systems, according to WHO, 'are defined as comprising all the organisations, institutions and resources that are devoted to producing actions principally aimed at improving, maintaining or restoring health' (2005: 2). Furthermore, health systems as interdependent constellations of organisations, institutions and resources are more than hospital and service delivery institutions, and more than the public sector. A health system 'includes the pyramid of health facilities and associated resources that deliver personal health services, and also non-personal health actions, for example anti-smoking, diet, and seat-belt campaigns' (WHO 2005: 6). Health systems also 'reflect their societies', and their development 'needs to be driven, not only by outcomes, but by shared values' and 'overall health goals: health gain, fairness, and responsiveness' (WHO 2005: 6). Progress towards these goals is linked to how well health systems carry out four key functions:

- stewardship (oversight and governance);
- financing (including revenue collection, fund pooling and purchasing);
- service delivery (for personal and non-personal health services);
- resource generation (investment in personnel as well as key inputs and technologies).

Stewardship

Stewardship is a broader concept than regulation and may be defined 'as the careful and responsible management of something entrusted to one's care. It involves influencing policies and actions in all the sectors that may affect population health' (WHO 2005: 9). The stewardship function is perhaps the most important function that governments have in respect of the health of their populations. It implies 'the ability to formulate strategic policy direction, to ensure good regulation and the tools for implementing it, and to provide the necessary intelligence on health system performance in order to ensure accountability and transparency' (WHO 2005: 9).

Stewardship is a complex function and embraces the following key issues and challenges:

- balancing multiple competing influences and demands while building coalitions and partnerships to achieve the principal health system objectives;
- establishing clear policy priorities;
- ensuring the necessary regulation of prices, professional practice, standards and so on;
- influencing the behaviour of the stakeholders involved through performance assessment and the provision of intelligence.

As WHO points out, the traditional function of many ministries of health is to provide services, not stewardship. Addressing the stewardship function involves major organisational changes. Whatever the differences between countries in their organisation of the stewardship function, 'every health system has to tackle the problems of designing, implementing, evaluating and reforming the organisations and institutions that facilitate the four key functions' (WHO 2005: 9). In many countries, including the UK, the notion of stewardship is under review as governments endeavour to be less centrally directive and more facilitative and enabling. This is especially evident in areas of public health policy, where politicians are anxious not to be seen as instruments of the 'nanny state'. With the thrust of policy in health and elsewhere on choice and individualism, telling people how to lead their lives is regarded as inconsistent and contradictory as well as being counterproductive.

Financing

Health system financing includes the mechanisms for collecting revenues, pooling these, and then distributing them among providers to improve health. In most health systems, these activities are discharged in such a way that they promote social solidarity and financial protection. Through such means, the health gap between rich and poor is reduced.

Service delivery

As has been noted already, health systems are often identified exclusively with service delivery and invariably with acute care in hospitals. Among the key issues in service delivery are: ensuring access to care among all social groups to reduce inequality, ensuring maximum population coverage, promoting patient safety, and understanding the impact of different service delivery strategies (such as public–private mix) on the health system.

Resource generation

Resources in the sense intended by WHO embrace not merely financial resources but also human resources, including universities and educational institutions, research centres and companies that produce

5

health care technologies such as medical devices and drug treatments. Investing in health systems to achieve the optimal balance of human resources and new technologies lies at the heart of resource generation.

According to WHO, examining the interaction between these four functions – stewardship, financing, service delivery and resource generation – permits an understanding of the determinants of health system performance and ultimately its impact on the health of a population. The stewardship function is the most important of the four functions because without it, the others cannot sensibly exist on their own. With the stewardship function firmly in place, the other functions can be organised appropriately to fulfil the shared values underpinning a health system.

With reference to the stewardship function as defined by WHO, a central challenge facing health systems in the 21st century is how to shift the emphasis from a preoccupation with secondary acute care services, largely provided in hospitals, to one that gives a higher priority to preventing ill-health and promoting health. Although infectious diseases have not been entirely conquered, and are making a reappearance in some cases, the significant pressures on health systems now come from non-communicable diseases, many of them – such as diabetes and heart disease – fuelled by the so-called 'diseases of comfort' such as obesity (Choi et al 2005). An ageing population has contributed to the demand for better integrated care in order to ensure the appropriate use of expensive hospital services. The priority in most advanced health systems is to control the demand for hospital beds and as far as possible treat and care for people in the community, either as an alternative to hospital care or as a means of reducing lengths of stay. It is not an especially new policy or radical departure in thinking, but is one that is nevertheless proving difficult to achieve.

Despite an expressed concern with health, most health systems in fact have become sickness services concerned chiefly with ill-health and disease. This bias was well described by Derek Wanless, a former banker commissioned by the UK government to advise on the future challenges facing the NHS over a 20-year period to 2020 and to come up with recommendations on what ought to be done to render it 'fit for purpose' in terms of tackling these challenges (Wanless 2002). Wanless was struck by the bias of the NHS to ill-health despite one of its founding principles being to promote the public's health. In fact, and notwithstanding important immunisation and vaccination programmes, the NHS for most of its 67 years has been preoccupied with treating people once they are ill. Various attempts to shift the emphasis have met with little success. In part this is due to powerful interests within the medical profession holding sway over which treatments get prioritised and funded. Following publication of a report by NHS England (2014), *The National Health Service Five Year Forward View*, the NHS is entering a period of considerable change centred on developing and testing new care models, initially in 29 vanguard sites, aimed at reducing the emphasis on traditional acute hospital care. Indeed, the Secretary of State for Health, Jeremy Hunt, who was reappointed to this position following the Conservative Party's slim victory in the May 2015 general election, has stated that his biggest priority is to transform care outside hospitals.

As already mentioned, although there is a comparative dimension to this book, its primary focus is on health policy in the United Kingdom and its evolution, especially in respect of developments since 2008 when the first edition appeared. The period in question covers the dying years of the last Labour government and the coalition government's tenure between 2010 and 2015. The position adopted is one articulated by Klein and Marmor (2006: 905), namely, 'the importance of context – institutional, ideological, and historical – in the understanding of policy making in modern polities'. At the same time, when the world is shrinking and innovations in information technology have accelerated the transfer of knowledge about developments in different countries, it is impossible to ignore entirely the comparative dimension. Rather, the issue is whether it helps or hinders understanding of what governments do and why.

Klein and Marmor consider three ways in which policy analysis might be improved through cross-national understanding. First, it can help to define more clearly what is on the policy agenda by reference to similar occurrences elsewhere. The issue of whether health systems are converging or diverging is considered below, but by providing a perspective or holding up a mirror, cross-national understanding can offer, as Klein and Marmor put it, 'explanatory insight or lesson drawing' (2006: 905).

A second application of cross-national understanding is to use it to test, or provide a check on, the adequacy of single-country accounts – what Klein and Marmor refer to as 'a defense against explanatory provincialism' (2006: 905). Similar or different configurations elsewhere can help develop a view about which particular features might be decisive, rather than simply present, in shaping policies or events.

A third approach in respect of valuing cross-national inquiry and understanding is to treat such experience as quasi-experiments. Here Klein and Marmor suggest that the purpose of these is 'to draw lessons about why some policies seem promising and doable, promising and impossible, or doable but not promising' (2006: 905). All three approaches appear in the comparative literature. The question is whether the promise such comparisons hold out for learning and lesson drawing is justified or not. The answer is a mixed one. Above all, it is important not to overstate global developments in health policy and, at the same time, not to understate the importance of context. With this proviso, the comparative dimension can enrich understanding of what may seem to be solely or exclusively national problems, and account for why ideas, which may be applied differently in different country contexts, have a cross-national appeal and resonance. In keeping with Klein and Marmor's view, it also offers a useful 'check on over-determined national explanations of why governments do what they do' (2006: 894).

Without in any way overlooking or oversimplifying the myriad of differences and subtleties that pervade, shape and ultimately characterise a country's health system, the key challenges facing these systems are broadly similar and are even described in similar terms. They have to do with the following features:

- financing of health care to ensure equity of access and provision – universal health coverage (UHC) is being promoted by WHO and other international bodies like the World Bank and Rockefeller Foundation as a pillar of sustainable development and global security that enables people to receive the health services they need without suffering financial hardship when paying for their care;
- the shifting roles of states and markets in health care with moves to reduce the size of the public sector and expand markets in the provision of health services;
- demographic trends pointing to ageing populations and the rapid rise of chronic and non-communicable diseases;
- the pandemic of diseases of affluence and lifestyle, notably obesity, alcohol misuse, mental ill-health and sexually transmitted infections;
- the shifting balance between primary and secondary care to give greater priority to the former;
- rebalancing health systems to give higher priority to health improvement and well-being (often referred to as public health) while viewing hospital services as a last resort when other upstream interventions have failed;
- health inequality and the widening health gap between rich and poor, which is occurring at a faster rate in some countries (such as the US and the UK) but is a feature of virtually all countries;
- giving public and patients greater voice and choice in their health care with, for example, the introduction of personal health budgets in the NHS in England to cover some aspects of long-term care.

Health systems: convergence or divergence?

An issue that preoccupies health policy analysts, especially those interested in comparative health systems, is whether the impact of globalisation and the international trade in management fads and fashions is resulting in countries converging as common solutions are applied to common problems (Blank and Burau 2004). Some analysts, such as Chernichovsky (1995), assert that despite the variety of health care systems – 27 in the European Union alone – the reforms of these systems have led to the emergence of what he terms a 'universal outline or paradigm' for health care financing, organisation and management. The paradigm cuts across ideological (public versus private) lines and across conceptual (market versus centrally planned) frameworks as it combines principles of public financing of health care (as enshrined in UHC) with principles of market competition applied to the organisation and management of the provision of health care. Much of this thinking has come directly from the World Bank, which since the 1990s has become more involved in health systems not only in developing countries but also in the countries making up the former Soviet Union in Central and Eastern Europe. There are also similarities in aspects of managing care between the UK and Australia, New Zealand, Canada and the US, although convergence is not envisaged. Simon Stevens, for example, appointed as NHS chief executive in April 2014 having previously been president for global health at the large US health insurance company, United Health, and before that health adviser to Tony Blair when Blair was prime minister, argues that while Britain and the US are in some ways moving in similar directions, they are doing so only up to a point (Stevens 2007).

In support of the convergence thesis is the globalisation of what has been termed 'new public management' (NPM) and its variants in 'Fordist' and 'post-Fordist' models. Chapter Two describes NPM in greater detail, but for present purposes it is enough to acknowledge the global reach of NPM and its association with public sector reform in areas such as health. James and Manning (1996) see NPM as an example of globalisation processes in public management that themselves have their roots in a set of pressures common across countries. Three pressures are especially acute: fiscal pressure (leading to a search for cost-containment measures in policy fields such as health), citizen pressure (resulting in more assertive and demanding citizens acting as consumers who wish to see rapid improvements in public services – a development to a large degree fuelled by governments and their political leaders preaching the virtues of choice and competition in health and health care), and the international promotion of reform ideas. This last pressure is particularly intriguing. James and Manning describe the phenomenon as follows: 'international management consultancy firms and public management organisations present the new forms to public managers as best practice' (1996: 144). Some of these firms, such as McKinsey's, have offices in more than 60 countries but no headquarters in the traditional sense, and provide a similar 'package' to different countries, thus spreading the new management concepts rapidly and with a degree of consistency previously unattainable. All these efforts are informed by a market-based ideology in which private sector practice is claimed to be superior and as providing a model for the transformation of allegedly underperforming, low-quality public services, and weak public sector management.

When these potent ideas are harnessed to the international community of management consultancies – no respecters of national boundaries or traditions – it is easy to see how an international policy culture of public sector management reform has developed. As a consequence, 'lesson drawing' is given a significant boost at a global level. Ideas and new forms of tackling policy puzzles and delivering health are communicated much more rapidly. If the globe is not converging, it is certainly contracting in respect of the transmission of, and access to, ideas and information, especially when filtered through conduits such as management consultancies. There is no doubt that enthusiasm among policy makers for external consultants has grown exponentially since around the mid-1990s (Craig 2006). The phenomenon is also part of the insidious growth of lobbying in countries' political systems, including in the US and UK, which has been termed a form of 'institutional corruption' (Draca 2014). Powerful and persistent lobbying, often on the part of large companies that are significant donors to particular political parties, can be corrosive of public service values. Later chapters will return to such matters. Meanwhile, we should return to the convergence/divergence issue and mention one further trend that may be making for greater convergence in a shrinking world.

In his epic study of war, peace and the course of history, Bobbitt (2003) examines the replacement of the nation state with the market state. This will happen (indeed, is already happening) because the nation state is unable to adapt to rapidly changing circumstances. As it increasingly loses its definition, the nation state will disappear. Indeed, Bobbitt alleges it may even come to be seen as an enemy of the people as a fragmenting public takes its various identities from largely non-national sensibilities. In such a context, the nation state is perceived as too rigid and confining. Globalisation is a key driver as it has undermined the collectivist values represented by the nation state and focused instead on the benefit of individuals. Given the declining membership of political parties and poor turnout at elections, there may be some substance to Bobbitt's thesis. But there are countervailing pressures, too, as evidenced in the resurgence of nationalism in countries like Scotland, the rise of left-wing parties in a number of European countries, and rise of right-wing parties in many countries, including England and France, in direct response to growing public unease over the impact of globalisation on jobs and high levels of immigration. However, different cultures will adapt and shape the market state in different and distinct ways so that in the UK, for example, a state-inflected market would probably develop, where government continued to maintain a strong presence through public financing of health care and ensured that a strong regulatory regime was in place.

Critics of the convergence thesis argue that it risks oversimplifying a complex reality that comprises divergence as well as convergence. So, in what follows, although it is suggested that a degree of convergence can be observed in respect of health system reform, which itself is associated with globalisation as a key driver for change, it would be a serious mistake and overly simplistic to overlook the very different contexts, cultures and political traditions in which such reform takes root and is modified and adapted in the process.

A framework for understanding the politics of health

To understand the evolution of health systems, and provide a structure for the discussion in subsequent chapters, it is helpful to employ a conceptual framework. Many such frameworks are available, and a useful and succinct review of the most prominent can be found in Baggott (2007). It is not the intention here to offer a similar review, but, instead, to draw on two frameworks from political science: first, Alford's (1975) classic study of health care politics in the US, and, second, Kingdon's (1986) multiple streams model. Before describing these frameworks in a little more detail, the importance of using a political science lens through which to study health policy merits justification. The role of politics in understanding complex, messy health systems is central. It is also why political science is uniquely well placed to explore its inner workings (Hunter 2015a and 2015b). Largely ignored and unappreciated, the discipline has much to offer those seeking a deeper understanding of current health systems, how they operate, and what needs to occur if they are to undergo effective and sustainable change. Politics is at the heart of all that happens in public policy and in complex systems, such as health, with their multiple levels of decision making and myriad groups of practitioners conducting power plays to achieve their ends (Marmor and Klein 2012).

Conceptualising health as political and as the product of political action has several practical implications when it comes to researching and comprehending complex health systems. In particular, the theories and insights offered by political science are well suited to providing a deeper understanding of the context of policy making (De Leeuw et al 2014). Political science deals with who gets what, when and how (Lasswell 1936) and public policy, including health, is therefore about politics resolving conflicts about resources, rights and morals (Klein and Marmor 2006). To make sense of health policy, analysts need to understand the frameworks underlying policy makers' choices, the institutions within, and through, which governments operate, and the interests of the different political actors involved. Political ideologies and institutions, the power of interest groups and lobbyists, media coverage (such as of a hospital closure) and public opinion all contribute to the definition and evolution of public policy.

Problems of implementation are often problems in developing political will and expertise to get things done. Far from being an unhelpful intrusion into the process of finding optimal solutions to complex problems, we need to put politics back into health. This was one of the challenges addressed in a recent report (Ottersen et al 2014) by The Lancet–University of Oslo Commission on Global Governance for Health, an independent academic panel set up to tackle reform in health-related global decision making. The Commission's report was the starting point for a Health Summit held at Durham University in November 2014 with the aim of putting politics back at the centre of global health (see special issue of *Public Health* on governance for health in a changing world, guest edited by Hunter, Schrecker and Alderslade 2015). Unless the social, commercial and political determinants of health are appreciated, the illusion will persist that technical fixes exist for global health problems and just need to be found. Far from seeking to remove politics from health, we need to re-politicise public policy in order to bring about change and improvement (Pfeffer 1992).

Let us return to the two political science frameworks mentioned above. Alford's framework is made up of three groups of structural interests – dominant professional interests, challenging corporate and managerial interests, and the repressed community interests.

The *dominant interests* comprise professional monopolists, principally doctors, whose values and sources of power are key drivers of health systems. They maintain their supremacy through underlying power generated by the social structure and by an ability to define the values of health care systems. By all accounts, the professional monopolists have been remarkably successful in influencing health policy and the design and operation of health systems.

The *challenging interests* are the corporate rationalisers, principally managers, whose power and authority have increased in recent years, thereby representing a challenge to the prevailing professional hegemony. The challenging interests have been concerned with improving efficiency and effectiveness as well as with quality of care.

Finally, there are the *repressed structural interests*, who comprise the public and who, for the most part, remain powerless in the face of the dominant and challenging interests. Recent changes in health systems have sought to accord a higher priority to user views and the voice of the public in shaping decisions and determining priorities.

Alford's framework has stood the test of time well and remains useful as a way of exploring and understanding the evolution of health systems from a political science perspective. The shifting relationship between the three groups of interests lies at the heart of the changing shape and fortunes of health systems and their respective politics. As several subsequent chapters endeavour to show, Alford's analysis helps to understand why reform fatigue has become a feature of health systems and why many of the desired changes have either, at best, not realised their full potential or, at worst, simply failed, only to be replaced by yet further change. The situation is described by Alford as one of 'dynamics without change'. Regardless of the precise nature of the various reforms of health systems that have been both proposed and implemented, they become absorbed into a system that is enormously resistant to change.

However, Alford goes further and characterises health system reformers as falling into one of two camps: 'market reformers', who hold state involvement in health care and bureaucratic complexity responsible for the ills apparent in health care systems; and 'bureaucratic reformers', who claim that the defects are all the fault of those who subscribe to markets and competition that obstruct the orderly planned provision of effective health care and have no place in medicine or health care. Again, the history of health systems is one that is marked by a constant oscillation between these reform models.

Kingdon's multiple streams, or organised anarchy model of public policy making, tease out the process's messiness, disjointedness, power asymmetry and sheer luck. The model comprises three streams that flow largely independently of one another. The *problem stream* focuses on a particular problem; the *political stream* is the governmental agenda of problems to be resolved; and the *policy stream* is the decision agenda from which a public policy may be selected. When these three streams converge they create 'windows' through which a public policy can result.

Both Alford's and Kingdon's frameworks are useful in illuminating health policy developments that are the subject of subsequent chapters. We shall therefore return to them from time to time in what follows.

Markets and medicine

The seemingly endless fascination with markets as a perceived solution to health system problems of inefficiency and poor performance has little basis in evidence. Or at least what limited evidence exists is vigorously contested. The upsurge of interest in evidence-based medicine has not been mirrored to quite the same degree in evidence-based policy. Evidence-*informed* policy may be the best outcome that can be hoped for but, for the most part and in keeping with the centrality of politics in public policy mentioned above, health system reforms are principally driven by a mix of ideologies and beliefs that then draw selectively on the evidence for support – more a case of policy-based evidence than evidence-based policy (Hunter 2009).

To illustrate the point, Evans (2005) asserts that the 'specious justifications' offered by the beneficiaries of private health systems (funding and provision) include the following: easing the financial burden on the public system, discouraging unnecessary and 'frivolous' care, and promoting greater efficiency through competition. Demonstrating that health policy is more about politics and power than evidence, Evans observes that these specious justifications have survived 'frequent logical or empirical refutation'. He concludes that the beneficiaries of what he terms 'privilege-preserving' funding arrangements 'are intellectual "zombies", constantly brought back to life by those whose interests they promote' (Evans 2005: 286). He goes on to note that these fundamental conflicts of interest around the funding of health care, and the extent to which it can or should be a universal and comprehensive public system, 'cannot be resolved by "fact and argument". These conflicts may go into remission, but they never disappear' (Evans 2005: 286).

In his essay on fads in management and health policy, Marmor supports Evans' critique, noting that 'the celebrations of markets and management had depleted faith in ordinary public administration' (Marmor 2004: 8). It is a view echoed by Sennett (2006) in his discourse on trust in politics and politicians. He suggests that the British New Labour government (1997-2010), acting as a consumer of policy, has done much to erode public trust in both the policies and politicians, resulting in a 'sour discontent' evident among people who sensed a government that was rudderless. 'Within the councils of government, the manufacture of ever-new policies appeared as an effort to learn from the actions previously taken; to the public, the policy factory seemed to indicate that government lacked commitment to any particular course of action' (Sennett 2006: 174). Policies on health, education and other sectors were spewed out 'with the same disenchanting effect' and in dramatic affirmation of Wildavsky's apt phrase 'doing better, feeling worse'. Sennett puts this restlessness and endless stream of policies down to a consumption mentality that fitted 'within the frame of new institutions' and was also evident in business, where short-term thinking prevailed. Perhaps the government had fallen victim to what an ex-McKinsey management consultant termed 'fad surfing', described as 'the practice of riding the crest of the latest management wave and then paddling out again just in time to ride the next one; always absorbing for managers and lucrative for consultants; frequently disastrous for organisations' (Shapiro 1996, quoted in Craig 2006: 235). And such policy restlessness is not confined to one particular political party. As leader of the opposition, for example, David Cameron insisted that there would be no further top-down reorganisation of the NHS, since the Conservative Party had come to appreciate that such change was often ineffective. As prime minister after the 2010 general election, however, he led a coalition government that proceeded to subject the NHS to arguably the most profound set of changes since its creation. The difficulties encountered in implementing these changes demonstrate the salience of Kingdon's multiple streams framework and the absence of alignment or convergence between them.

The history of the NHS over most of its 67 years is marked by a series of struggles. On the one side are those who are opposed to what they consider to be an outdated form of nationalised health care and who insist that a more decentralised and market-led health system is what people want and expect in the 21st century (the market reformers to whom Alford refers). On the other side are those who continue to hold to the view that, for all its imperfections, there really is no markedly better system of health care if the aim is low cost and equitable access to care as well as a health service that is based on need and not on ability to pay (Alford's bureaucratic reformers).

Critics of the NHS accuse it of being over-centralised and sclerotic, lacking responsiveness to patient needs, and too readily becoming the plaything of politicians who are seemingly unable to stop meddling with it. The constant reorganisations of the NHS, the critics assert, bear testimony to these fundamental flaws in its conception and management. Supporters of the NHS, on the other hand, while accepting that there are weaknesses with the high degree of political interference – which can be dysfunctional, resulting in what has been termed the politicisation of managers – claim it is not the model itself that is defective or flawed but the way in which it has developed and become distorted by politicians masquerading as micro-managers. They point to the Spanish NHS, which is characterised by a high level of devolution to semi-autonomous regional governments. This reflects a political system that is decentralised in contrast to the NHS in the UK, which until recently was the most centralised in Western Europe and probably far beyond. The arrival of political devolution in 1999 has resulted in increasing divergence in respect of health policy across the four countries making up the UK. The differences are especially marked between England and Scotland, where there has been greater resistance to market-style solutions. Following the Scottish National Party's (SNP) landslide victory at the 2015 general election when it won 53 of the 56 Scottish seats, further powers will be devolved to the Scottish parliament in Edinburgh. There is also the prospect of a further referendum on independence after the September 2014 vote found in favour of those opposing independence. The pro-independence vote was nevertheless significant and led to an unforeseen surge of support for the SNP that led to Labour's virtual demise in Scotland (holding just one seat) at the general election.

Meanwhile, the English state, with a population of around 48 million people, remains highly centralised, although changes may be afoot with the Conservative government's enthusiasm for the 'Northern Powerhouse' initiative that will initially devolve responsibility for large parts of the public sector, including the NHS, to Greater Manchester and to a new elected regional partnership board (Association of Greater Manchester Authorities 2015). Known as Devo Manc, this move has triggered enthusiasm elsewhere in England for similar devolved arrangements although not all the schemes being considered include health. If this new-found enthusiasm for devolving power proves popular, the way public services are organised and led could change significantly, with the locus of power to be found not centrally but locally. This could result in greater diversity and variation in provision and different choices being made as to the degree to which services are subjected to market forces and the exercise of personal choice. Perhaps for this reason, the secretary of state for health is determined to retain reserve powers to overturn decisions affecting the NHS of which he or see disapproves (Paine 2015). This is because of a tension between the 'national' in NHS and 'local' in local government. In practice, therefore, it may be more a case of delegated rather than devolved powers over health care.

One of the principal architects of market forces in health care systems is Alain Enthoven; his influence over the internal market reforms ushered in by the Conservative government in the early 1990s was considerable, even if it was more by luck than design as Enthoven himself acknowledged. His booklet, *Reflections on the Management of the National Health Service* (1985), published by Nuffield Provincial Hospitals Trust, found its way onto the reading list of government ministers, including the then prime minister, Margaret Thatcher. By market forces Enthoven means 'significant responsible consumer choice among providers, and providers who gain their incomes from serving the consumers who chose them' (2002: 5). He is motivated by a desire to create incentives for providers to innovate in ways that improve outcomes, including patient satisfaction, and reduce costs.

Reflecting some years later on his experience in reforming the NHS, at a time when New Labour was busy reintroducing market forces into health care having spent its first few years insisting it had abolished them, Enthoven notes that New Labour, while claiming to do something different, in fact built on and extended the Thatcher reforms. The government retained the purchaser–provider split and the NHS hospital trust idea. Indeed, it went further and introduced foundation trusts whereby hospitals that passed certain tests in respect of possessing robust business plans could become independent not-for-profit institutions. Finally, the government also permitted contracting with hospitals regardless of whether they were public, private or voluntary. Through such means, the potential exists for the NHS to be recast as a purchaser on behalf of patients, fully committed to the interests of patients rather than being captive to powerful provider interests. Indeed, this was the purpose of the coalition government's 2013 NHS reforms, which began soon after its election in May 2010. Liberating the patient was the strapline for the changes, although over time, this focus got lost amid the complexity of the organisational changes introduced.

Enthoven's scepticism that it will be possible to change 'deeply ingrained habits' acquired over many decades may have been proved well founded. He poses the following questions:'Will the government be able to let go? Will ministers be able to resist responding to every problem with a blizzard of new directives? Will politicians be able to resist making the details of health care into political issues?' (2002: 8). The answer to these questions, on the basis of all the evidence since Enthoven wrote these words, is an unequivocal 'no'. It has not so far proved possible for ministers to let go and exercise a self-denying ordinance when problems arise. A good example is hospital-acquired infection, which has been rising in the UK at a faster rate than in other countries. Whenever there is a media scare about the state of dirty hospitals and the deaths of patients from *c. difficile* or MRSA, ministers feel compelled to announce a new target or initiative aimed at eradicating the problem. They do so at the same time as preaching the virtues of local decision making and reduced central control.

Those critical of market forces in health care regard markets as beset by what is termed 'market failure', including uncertainty, moral hazard, adverse selection and asymmetry of information. They also adhere to a value system that contends that nobody should go without necessary care for lack of ability to pay. As Enthoven himself concedes, 'this makes creation of a market in health care that drives improvement a particularly complex undertaking' (2002: 13). As ever, the devil is in the detail. Particular attention must be given to what can and cannot be left to the market, with partial implementation likely to end in failure. Much of the criticism of the coalition government's NHS changes, as we shall see in later chapters, concerns the issue of markets and competition and their place in health.

One of Enthoven's more important and insightful reflections seems to go to the heart of the politics of health care reform. In a crucial passage he observes that just because something is done in the private sector does not mean that rational economic incentives will always apply. Conversely, the fact that something is in the public sector does not necessarily mean that such incentives do not apply. The reality is more complicated, as the experience of the US shows, where, according to Enthoven, it is the public sector employers who have performed best in implementing rational economic structures for employee health care. This observation might also be true of Sweden, where health care reform has centred on making publicly operated institutions more efficient and able to respond to economic incentives (Saltman and Bergman 2005).

The crucial point about Enthoven's caveat concerning market forces and the private sector is that getting the conditions and detail right is precisely what governments are notoriously bad at doing. The point is well made by Kettl when he says that:

> Despite the enthusiasm for entrepreneurial government and privatisation, the most egregious tales of waste, fraud, and abuse in government programs have often involved greedy,

> corrupt, and often criminal activity by the government's private partners – and *weak government management to detect and correct these problems*. (Kettl 1993: 5, emphasis added)

The government's relationships with the private sector in health as elsewhere require what Kettl calls 'aggressive management by a strong, competent government' (1993: 6). Competition might advance efficiency but not always and not automatically. Paradoxically, the government's growing reliance on the private sector is weakening its capacity to manage public–private partnerships, since the expertise required has been lost. The danger then is that having sought diversity of provision with the private sector competing with publicly operated institutions it becomes difficult if not impossible effectively to regulate the new marketplace that has been created. It begins to take on a life of its own. As Evans (2005) put it, once the genie is out of the bottle it cannot be put back in. Markets do not automatically self-regulate and to assume otherwise is naive in the extreme. Moreover, functions often end up in the public sector for good reason. Goals are complex, varied and sometimes conflicting. It is up to the political process to negotiate an acceptable compromise for the optimal way forward. Often there is no final outcome but simply a series of negotiated settlements.

The irony is that market failures or imperfections are the principal justification for government intervention in areas such as health care. Yet (regardless, it seems, of which party, or combination of parties in the case of the coalition, is in charge) much of the UK government's health system reform programme is not so much new as a case of 'back to the future', since the mixed economy of care favoured harks back to the pre-NHS arrangements. But it was precisely because those arrangements were of such greatly varying quality, and because variations in access to treatment were so wide and increasingly unacceptable, that the NHS was established in 1948. Given that market imperfections are a feature of all sectors, only government can assert strong control over markets. However, unless government possesses the requisite political will and skills, it will fail to act and market failure will go unchallenged.

As the above discussion of public services and markets demonstrates, the issues are not primarily ones of fact or logic or even evidence. History, culture, tradition, values and above all politics count for more in shaping the design of health care systems and in determining their progress. As the social historian and health policy analyst Rosemary Stevens argues, 'decisions on many aspects of medical resources are political and economic: the result of social decisions rather than of individual judgement, or even the judgement of physicians ...' (2007: 157). It seems the 18th-century pathologist-turned-anthropologist, Rudolf Virchow, was right when he asserted that 'medicine is a social science and politics nothing but medicine on a grand scale' (quoted in Miller 1973: v).

Plan of book

Following this introductory chapter, Chapter Two provides a broad overview of how health systems in a variety of contexts are responding to the broadly similar challenges they face through a combination of managerialism and markets, which come together in the idea of new public management and its more recent variants. It sets the scene for the subsequent four chapters and considers why changes that are heralded as pioneering, and are viewed as putting health services on a new and different footing, often fail to live up to expectations and are then criticised for having been 'oversold'.

The themes briefly reviewed above form the basis for much of what follows in Chapters Three to Six. As mentioned at the start of the chapter, much of the book is structured around four closely interconnected and interlocking themes or policy cleavages. To recap briefly, they are:

- the balance between health care and health;
- the funding and organisation of health care systems with their mix of public and private arrangements;
- the ways in which health systems prioritise or ration health care;

- the growing commodification of health as a market-style consumer good in which notions of choice and competition vie with notions of collectivism and solidarity.

Chapters Three to Six each deal with one of the four topics, or policy cleavages, listed above and review the competing arguments surrounding them. Given the interlocking nature of the themes that make up these chapters, there is inevitably some repetition, but, as far as possible, it has been kept to a minimum.

Chapter Three looks at the wider public health debate that is gathering pace in many countries that have concluded that merely funding health systems as presently configured is unsustainable and that a paradigm shift to a health, as distinct from ill-health or sickness, society is overdue. A starting point for this debate is that most of the gains in population health have less to do with health care services than they do with factors and policies outside health care. This is not to deny that health services have an important contribution to make to improved health, but they are insufficient on their own and in the absence of an ecological approach to health that recognises the importance of structural determinants on health. Furthermore, many of the growing pressures on acute care services arise from lifestyle-related illnesses and conditions that are avoidable. Following the UK coalition government's Health and Social Care Act 2012, the lead for public health in England was transferred from the NHS to local government in an effort to give it a higher priority. The chapter draws on research led by the author and colleagues into the new public health system.

Chapter Four examines the evolution of health reform and the three phases it has passed through, as demonstrated by developments in the UK. The UK experience provides a good case study of health care reorganisation because it has been subjected to successive, and almost continuous, waves of reform since the mid-1970s. The most recent of these followed the coalition government's determination to reform the NHS from 2013 in the face of considerable professional and public opposition. Because of the highly centralised nature of the NHS, policy makers can change its structure and the incentives that operate within it in an instant or on a whim. At least, they can give the *illusion* of change – an important distinction. In a complex undertaking employing over one million people, the reality of implementing change is uncertain and far from straightforward, and is by no means guaranteed in the manner often assumed through ministerial diktat. This was very much the case with regard to the changes put forward by the coalition government.

Chapter Five considers rationing and priority setting in health care and reviews how these are being tackled. Whereas rationing was on every policy maker's lips a decade or so ago, rather less was heard about it during the 1990s and 2000s. But with austerity policies being implemented in many countries following the financial crash in 2008–10, health budgets are being squeezed and talk of rationing services is back on the agenda. In the UK, the National Institute for Health and Care Excellence (NICE), and its equivalent in Scotland, the Scottish Intercollegiate Guidelines Network (SIGN), have largely kept the dreaded 'r' word (rationing) that strikes fear into the hearts of politicians off the agenda. But in introducing the Cancer Drugs Fund in 2010, the coalition government, however unintentionally, undermined NICE's primary purpose. There are also issues about the extent to which NICE guidance is implemented. This chapter considers these and other issues involving the media and influence of Big Pharma on policy. 'Big Pharma' refers to the global drug lobby made up of representatives from the large pharmaceutical companies to influence governments, the media and sometimes patient groups in favour of the pharmaceutical industry and its products (Goldacre 2012).

Chapter Six probes a little deeper in respect of two components of the market-style changes under way in many health systems – choice and competition. It is widely believed by reformers that without choice and competition, even within publicly funded and organised health systems, there can be no guarantee of services that are responsive to patients' wishes, or efficient and effective in terms of quality. Other policy instruments available to incentivise change include setting targets and managing performance through inspection and regulation, but these are seen as having defects and are not regarded as an effective substitute for choice and competition, although these may proceed in tandem, which can add to the complexity evident in health systems. In the NHS in England, there have been moves to introduce personal health budgets to give patients more control over the management of their health including appropriate treatments for medical conditions. A similar model has been used in social care settings for some years.

Finally, Chapter Seven provides an assessment of the current state of the health debate, drawing together some of the key elements of the policy cleavages considered in the preceding chapters. It returns to the relevance and importance of Alford's and Kingdon's frameworks and their political analysis perspective as aids to understanding health systems and how they discharge the four key functions of stewardship, financing, service delivery, and resource generation as these are played out in contemporary health debates about health system reform. These debates include choice and competition, priorities and rationing, and health as distinct from health care. The chapter also offers an alternative approach to the pervasive influence of markets and competition in health system reform to illustrate its essentially political nature – one that is far from being evidence-based.

It seems only fair to the reader to declare my own values and biases at the outset of this book. While endeavouring to present the principal arguments and contrasting views in an even-handed and balanced manner, the book nevertheless adopts a clear position in respect of each of the policy cleavages reviewed. It is not, and makes no pretence to be, an impartial text, assuming there is such a thing in the first place – which is doubtful. Running through the book is a belief in the essential values and ethos of the UK NHS and a frustration that many of the policy changes inflicted upon it over the past 18 years or so have been misconceived and are likely to fail, thereby paving the way for a possible replacement of the NHS in all but name. In particular, the frustration is with the dominant political values that appear to inform contemporary health policy reform, and the tendency to ignore or overlook possible alternative reform strategies that might not only be preferable but have an equal or better chance of success.

TWO

Meeting the health system challenges

Introduction

In Chapter One, the value of a comparative approach in describing and understanding health systems was mentioned albeit with an acknowledgement of the limitations of such an approach and the tendency to overlook key cultural and historical differences between countries and their health systems. These cultural and historical factors often play a major role in the way those systems function regardless of the details of their funding and organisation. Through making comparisons it is possible to identify both commonalities and differences. The notion of convergence in an increasingly globalised world was also considered in Chapter One. Whatever the value, and reality, of the convergence thesis, a variety of health systems exists and important differences remain. This chapter describes the principal features of health systems and explores the powerful appeal of managerialism and markets to provide an overall context against which to consider the various policy cleavages that occupy the rest of the book.

Types of health system

In this section, we describe the various types and key features of health systems. The principal types are set out in Box 2.1.

Box 2.1: Types of health care system

Private insurance   Social insurance   National health service

Free market system   -------------   Government monopoly

The US 'non-system' of health comes closest to the free market system, while, at least until recently, the UK's NHS comes closest to a system representing a government monopoly at the other extreme. Box 2.2 shows the principal types of funding.

Box 2.2: Types of funding

- Direct tax/general revenues
- Social or state insurance
- Private insurance
- Direct payment by users

The UK's NHS is an example of a health system funded principally by direct taxation, although there are user charges for some groups of patients in the form of prescription charges. However, these charges only apply to England and, since devolution, no longer apply in Wales and Scotland. Most Western European health systems are funded through a method of social insurance combined with opt-outs so that people can take out private insurance. An extensive review of social insurance schemes as part of a wider review of NHS financing, conducted in 2002 (Wanless 2002), concluded that for the NHS there should be no change in the principle of funding health care through general taxation. However, critics of the NHS and its alleged centralised and heavily politicised structure favour a social insurance system on the grounds that this would allow the NHS to free itself of political interference and an overbearing form of central control. There is no certainty that such an outcome would occur and that what may work in one system can simply be imported to another, regardless of its particular context and features. It is important to appreciate the historical, economic, social and political influences that combine to determine the precise design and operation of a country's health system. In the absence of such an appreciation, the result may be unforeseen and unintended consequences. In any event, when it comes to the funding of health systems, the Economist Intelligence Unit (2015) concluded that the NHS was 'an incredibly lean and efficient health service compared with just about every other industrialised country'. And in its 2014 update of its analysis of the performance of 11 countries, the Commonwealth Fund (Davis et al 2014) ranked the UK's health system first (discussed in more detail later in the chapter). As Street (2015) has argued, social insurance models are typified by high administrative costs, over-treatment and over-pricing. Compared with European health systems funded by social insurance, the UK spends the least by far – 9.1% of GDP (amounting to £112 billion a year). In France, the proportion of GDP spent on health is 11.7%, in Switzerland it is 11.5% and in Germany it is 11.3%. The Netherlands spends 12.9% of its GDP on health.

The types of political culture within which different types of health system are located are listed in Box 2.3.

Box 2.3: Political cultures relating to different health systems

Communitarian	Egalitarian	Individualistic
Germany	Sweden	USA
Netherlands	New Zealand	Australia
Japan	UK	Singapore

Few countries fit neatly into one or other column, but an attempt has been made to locate them in keeping with their predominant characteristics. For example, although the UK is regarded as egalitarian as a result of its post-World War II welfare state, the country has some of the most pronounced health inequalities between social groups, with the health gap widening (Dowler and Spencer 2007a; Dunnell 2008; Office for National Statistics 2008). In its comparison of 11 health systems, the Commonwealth Fund (Davis et al 2014) scores the UK high on overall equity with small differences between lower- and higher-income adults on most measures. But the UK lags notably on health outcomes, coming just ahead of the US. Three outcome indicators were used – mortality amenable to medical care, infant mortality, and healthy life expectancy at age 60. The UK's poor score reflects a complex mix of factors, but high among them is the growing health gap between social groups, noted by Marmot in his review of how best to tackle inequalities in health (Marmot 2010), and a continuing failure to give sufficient priority to improving population health (see Chapter Three).

Finally, in describing health systems, the mix of public–private funding and provision is of interest and this is depicted in Box 2.4. In seeking to reform their systems, countries are faced with few options when it comes to funding health care. Indeed, in order to control cost inflation in health care, countries have generally favoured increased public control of funding. Most reform initiatives tend to focus on the mix of provision, with a growing emphasis on private provision (including for-profit and not-for-profit) to stimulate competition in the belief that this improves efficiency and raises the quality of care. As Box 2.4 shows, the UK is high in respect of both public funding and public provision, although in respect of the latter, the mix is changing in favour of greater pluralism and diversity with active encouragement being given to for-profit and not-for-profit providers, including mutual and other forms of social enterprise. As later chapters will show, these developments began in earnest under the three Labour governments between 1997 and 2010 and were pursued with greater vigour by the coalition government between 2010 and 2014, culminating in the Health and Social Care Act 2012 (see Chapter Four).

Box 2.4: Public control of funding and provision of health care

	Public control of provision		
	High	Middle	Low
Public control of funding — High	UK Sweden		Japan Netherlands
Middle	Australia New Zealand	Germany	
Low	Singapore		United States

Health systems having been established, the politics of health then revolve around the competing goals of health care. These are:

- equity/access
- quality
- cost containment (efficiency).

No country has established a perfect balance between this so-called three-legged stool; the endless, and often restless, search for one dominates the health debate. It also demonstrates the essentially political nature of the discourse in health systems even if this is often disguised and becomes obfuscated by reducing issues and policy puzzles to seemingly technocratic matters and resorting to a particular form of managerialism to achieve results.

In the UK, with the advent of political devolution in 1999, there is – at least at one level – evidence of growing divergence between the four countries, with Wales and Scotland in particular developing their own distinctive health systems (for further details about the four health systems see the European Observatory on Health Systems and

Policies Health Systems in Transition reports on the UK – Boyle 2011; Longley et al 2012; Steel and Cylus 2012; O'Neill et al 2012). When it comes to financing, there is virtually no difference across the UK, apart from prescription charges, which still apply in England but have been abolished in Wales and Scotland. In terms of structure and approaches to market-style changes, there are marked differences, with England favouring moves towards a mixed economy of care and displaying a constant preoccupation with structural changes that have not been replicated elsewhere. This is especially evident in Scotland, where the Scottish National Party (SNP) has positioned itself to the left of the Labour Party on social policy and public sector reform issues. Having won 53 of the 56 seats in Scotland, the SNP is now intent on winning further devolved powers and is determined to pursue a very different programme of social democratic change from that being pursued in England following the Conservative Party's unexpected election win in May 2015.

When it comes to targets to reduce waiting lists and times, and improve access to care, the approach adopted in England has been much tougher and unrelenting than elsewhere. Some observers claim that such an approach has worked to England's advantage because waiting lists are lower and care more efficient (Bevan and Hood 2006). But others argue that even if there is evidence that targets work in improving performance, merely reducing waiting lists says nothing about the quality of care received or outcomes (Propper et al 2008). Such arguments, however, ignore the acknowledgement of widespread cheating, or 'gaming', to meet nationally imposed targets, which suggests that perhaps not all is as it seems (Seddon 2003). After all, if a chief executive's career is on the line for failing to meet a target, whatever it takes to meet the target will be sanctioned. It is a perfectly rational response under the circumstances. Failure is not an option.

Returning to the evidence of intra-UK differences, policy makers in Wales and Scotland argue that they have established different priorities that are relevant to, and directed towards, their respective health systems. In both countries, there has been a greater emphasis on public health and on tackling health inequality. However, it remains to be seen whether such differences in emphasis are substantive or merely rhetorical (Smith et al 2008). It is also important to appreciate, too, but all too easy to forget in the preoccupation with difference and devolved arrangements, that Wales and Scotland do not exist in sealed compartments. They remain intimately bound up with the UK and there is much movement of personnel between the four health systems within the UK, who bring with them their particular experience acquired in another setting, just as there is movement of individuals for personal and family reasons. Pressures for convergence rather than divergence within the UK therefore remain powerful despite devolution and the rise of those pressing for independence in Scotland both prior to the referendum held in September 2014 and since, following the surge in support for the SNP, and the opportunities presented by their election victory to do things differently.

International league tables and international comparisons of health systems make for interesting conversations in pubs and at dinner tables. But it is questionable how valuable they really are; often the sources of such comparisons need to be viewed with caution and a fair degree of scepticism. The Commonwealth Fund survey (Davis et al 2007) has been criticised for its methodology, which, it is claimed, distorts its conclusions concerning the performance of the British NHS. For instance, a study by the think tank, Civitas, calls the survey a 'caricature' of health system performance that 'distorts proper analysis by ranking entire health systems on what are, quite frankly, inadequate measures' (Gubb 2007: 25). However, it is important to put the Commonwealth Fund's international comparative performance of health care in perspective. First, it is principally aimed at showing how performance has improved or deteriorated over time in the US (Davis et al 2007). Second, the Fund acknowledges that any attempt to assess the relative performance of countries has inherent limitations. Among these are the fact that assessments of health system performance are likely to be affected by the experiences and expectations of patients and physicians, and that these may well differ by country and culture. Having said that, the Commonwealth Fund's work, which started in 2004 with subsequent editions appearing in 2006, 2007, 2010 and 2014, has been extensively and approvingly cited by government ministers and senior policy advisers and managers. The Fund is a highly respected and well regarded authority.

In its 2014 update, the Fund looked at the comparative performance of the health systems in 11 countries representing a range of health system types as described above. The countries, in alphabetical order, are:

- Australia
- Canada
- France
- Germany
- Netherlands
- New Zealand
- Norway
- Sweden
- Switzerland
- United Kingdom
- United States.

In each country, an assessment of performance was made covering six categories. The categories are:

- quality of care
- access to care
- efficiency of health system
- equity of health system
- ability to ensure long, healthy and productive lives.

In terms of the key findings reported, the US ranks last of the 11 nations – as it did in all of the earlier surveys since 2004 – failing to achieve better health outcomes than the other countries in the survey and coming last on dimensions of access, efficiency, equity and healthy lives. The UK, on the other hand, continues to demonstrate superior performance in all dimensions with the exception of healthy lives, followed by Switzerland and Sweden. The most notable way in which the US has differed from other countries, until the introduction of the Affordable Care Act in 2010 that will help extend health insurance coverage to an estimated 26 million previously uninsured Americans, has been the absence of universal health insurance coverage. It is not surprising, therefore, that the US performs significantly worse than other countries on measures of access to care and equity in health care between populations with above-average and below-average incomes. The area where the US health care system performs best is preventive care, an area that has been monitored closely for over a decade by managed care plans whose success comes from keeping people out of expensive hospital care. Despite this, the survey notes that the US scores particularly poorly on its ability to promote healthy lives. This may not be so surprising as the US is a world leader in rapidly rising rates of obesity among adults and children, principally the result of its fast-food culture and lack of exercise among its population (Kawachi 2007).

The survey concludes that in all countries there is room for improvement. But it also notes that all the countries spend considerably less than the US on health care per person and as a percentage of gross domestic product (US per capita spending on health is more than double the average among industrialised nations belonging to the Organisation for Economic Co-operation and Development). The US could therefore 'do much better in achieving better value for the nation's substantial investment in health' (Davis et al 2007: viii).

Seasoned observers of international health systems will not be surprised at these findings or at their persistence over time. But what may surprise readers is that despite the generally poor performance of the US health system (or 'non-system', since there is no single system as such but a fragmented, uncoordinated patchwork of services), it continues to attract considerable interest from health system reformers in other countries, who regard the US as a repository of innovation and successful initiatives demonstrating the important, and largely benign, influence of markets in health care. Such a contradictory response to the US health 'system' and its generally poor performance may seem somewhat mystifying. Seeking to explain it would take us far beyond the purposes and limits of this book. However, the authors of the

35

Commonwealth Fund survey suggest that the US could learn from innovations in other countries, not something that comes naturally to those running health care in the US. As the report states: 'Like the queen in the "Snow White" fairy tale, Americans often look only at their own reflection in the mirror – failing to include international experience in assessments of the health care system' (Davis et al 2007: 1). This lacuna is an example of the power of values and culture over how not just health policy but all public policy gets conceived and shaped and why there are strict limits on how far international comparisons are useful.

The Commonwealth Fund comparison noted the following features of the UK's NHS:

- it makes more use of nurses in routine care management of sicker adults;
- it makes more use of multidisciplinary teams in primary care;
- it scores relatively poorly in measures concerning patient centred care;
- it is more likely to set targets for clinical performance;
- it allows speedier access to a doctor than in the US;
- it has better out of hours access than the US;
- a UK resident with above-average income is much more likely to have their blood pressure checked than someone with below-average income – the reverse is true in the US.

What can sensibly be said about this mix of features is not obvious; they probably have their roots in history and custom and practice for which there may be no rational explanation. However, the picture that does emerge is that for all the criticism levelled at it within the UK, the NHS is by no means bankrupt as a system. Nor, at nearly 68 years of age, has it had its day, as some of its critics and sections of the media like to believe. Even the Civitas report (Gubb 2007) concedes that avoidable mortality from the biggest killers – circulatory disease and cancer – has improved quite markedly between 1999 and 2005 in England and Wales. It concludes that NHS performance since 1999 'looks fairly impressive in the international context', with above average improvements in the biggest killers 'compared with other European countries of comparable development' (Gubb 2007: 24). Nevertheless, despite the improvements, it expresses concern that avoidable mortality rates remain comparatively very high. However, establishing the causes of these is complex and it may be that the NHS – or indeed any health care system – on its own can do little if it is changing lifestyles that are largely responsible for much of the problem. As already mentioned, the obesity 'epidemic' may be a major cause of the increase in certain diseases along with other lifestyle-related conditions such as alcohol misuse. In any event, given that there is no such thing as a perfect health system anywhere in the world, the UK's NHS would still appear to have much to commend it. In common with other systems, it wrestles with some deep-seated and persistent dilemmas and challenges that together constitute what might be termed the health debate and in doing so there is evidence of both failures and achievements.

Meeting the challenges facing health

In meeting the various challenges that comprise the health debate, and which were briefly described in Chapter One, modern health systems have pursued a number of reform strategies over the past 50 years or so, with the pace quickening since the 1980s. Since then, the NHS has been subjected to unrelenting continuous change in its architecture and policy environment. Most of the various reforms can be analysed and best understood by reference to Alford's framework of dominant (medical profession), challenging (management and managers) and repressed (the public) structural interests introduced in the previous chapter. The playing out of these structural interests has occurred alongside another, and not unrelated, struggle, also noted by Alford, namely, that between market-style reformers on the one hand and bureaucratic reformers on the other.

Despite the preoccupation among policy makers with health system reform, radical change is rarely a serious option – at least not in practice, regardless of the promises policy makers may make in their rhetoric.

When the Conservative government began toying with market-style reforms of the British NHS in the early 1990s, its efforts proved to be less far-reaching than many wished or initially intended, and the government pulled back from giving free rein to the market, much to the regret of some observers who were keen to test the role of markets in health care and believed they had a place by incentivising providers to perform differently (Le Grand 2007). The reason was entirely political. Since the NHS is widely regarded by the public as a cherished institution, akin perhaps to the BBC, no government dare risk its own existence by tampering with the NHS in a way that might put its very survival at stake. An exception to this conventional wisdom was the 2010 coalition government's unprecedented and ambitious plans for the NHS in England led by the then Secretary of State for Health, Andrew Lansley. Chapter Four covers this puzzling episode in health policy in greater depth, but suffice to say here that in opposition, the Conservative Party leader, David Cameron, went on record stating that under his watch there would be no further top-down reforms of the NHS since they did not work.

Some years earlier, for reasons that are not entirely clear and that certainly contradicted the government's own reform rhetoric at the time, the New Labour government that succeeded the Conservatives in 1997 went much further in introducing market-style mechanisms into the NHS. Indeed, the journey along this path continued under the coalition government, which defended its actions by arguing that they were in keeping with the direction already set by New Labour.. However, regardless of the prevailing political situation in any particular country, it seems generally to be the case that major path-breaking change is infrequent and very much the exception. Path dependence would appear to be the norm, which contends that policy options are limited by facts and vested interests on the ground – institutional structures and the consequences of past decisions all conspire to constrain the ability of policy makers to strike out in wholly new directions (Oliver and Mossialos 2005). While this is generally true, there are also occasions when the notion of 'punctured equilibrium' may apply, that is, a change that has profound and far-reaching impacts and implications (Gould 1990). A good example of this phenomenon is the introduction of the NHS itself in 1948, while a more recent example might be political devolution within the UK in the late 1990s, ushering in elected assemblies in Wales and Northern Ireland, and a parliament in Scotland. In Scotland, Labour was narrowly defeated by the SNP in the May 2007 election with the result that policy divergence, already a feature, is likely to grow. Given the SNP's success in governing, both in a minority government and as the majority party in Scotland, not to mention its impressive gains in the 2015 UK general election, further devolved powers may see greater policy divergence occurring. But of course, as noted earlier, there are constraints operating that can limit the degree of radical change possible and make path dependence a more likely driver of what happens regardless of the rhetoric surrounding new policy initiatives.

Not all changes result in a sharp departure from the past, despite a desire on the part of the reformer to bring about such an outcome or at least to present it as such. An example is New Labour's attempt to reform the NHS, especially in the later years of Tony Blair's premiership from around 2002. The results proved to be far less significant or impressive than the rhetoric accompanying them would suggest. As any change management text will state, the chances of ensuring that successful implementation occurs are seriously impaired if those working on the front line do not embrace the changes and seek to contest, or undermine, them. The Blair government ignored this wise counsel to its cost, as did the coalition government in 2010 when it launched its own NHS upheaval. A feature of the most recent changes in the NHS in England is that the key professions in the NHS have been disengaged from the reform process. Yet, as the work of Lipsky (1980) on street-level bureaucrats suggests, the discretion and power exercised by those on the front line may prove instrumental in determining the success or failure of a policy or set of structural changes.

Blair thought he could bypass the medical profession, regarding it as the major source of the problem rather than at least part of the solution. And for a time he was able to do so. Indeed, one reason for resorting to the private health care sector and encouraging private companies to provide services in direct competition with the NHS, primarily in the form of independent sector treatment centres (see Chapter Four), was to avoid dependence on – and being held to ransom by – the monopoly position enjoyed by the NHS. In so doing, the aim was to encourage the NHS to raise its game when confronted with competition on its local patch. But the experiment cannot be said to have been a resounding success; one of its consequences has been a serious lowering of morale among the workforce and a widespread perception among staff and public that despite unprecedented levels of investment in the NHS between 2002 and 2008, averaging annual growth of 7.4% over the five years with spending rising by nearly 50%, the service remains a poor performer in terms of overall productivity (Wanless et al 2007). Part of the reason for this has been placed on the degree and extent of organisational change, which 'has been costly, not just financially but in terms of disruption, loss of experienced staff and changes in working relationships both within the NHS and with external organisations' (Wanless et al 2007: xxvii). Presumably it was comments such as this that underlay David Cameron's promise not to inflict further top-down reorganisation on the NHS, which makes doubly perplexing the reason why he reneged on it so soon after entering office.

Other reasons for low staff morale and poor performance lie in successive governments' obsession with centrally imposed targets as a means of achieving change (Seddon 2003). To meet its targets, the New Labour government through most of the 2000s sought to increase capacity and did so by investing significant new resources. The expectation was that by investing more, the system would produce more and do more work. But this rather assumes that the system was already functioning optimally and without waste or inefficiencies. Otherwise, adding resources to a wasteful system simply compounds the inefficiency – a case of putting good money after bad. Seddon's argument is that the targets imposed by government 'are themselves a major cause of waste, consuming people's time in artificial activity and, worse, deflecting their attention from what they ought to be doing' (Seddon 2003: 208). For Seddon and proponents of lean thinking, the critical thing is for managers to manage the overall flow of work rather than functions within it. A target-based approach tends to focus on functions while ignoring the whole system and the flow of work within it.

If there is a consistent theme running through health system reform of an absence of major, path-breaking change, with policy options limited by what is feasible on the ground with the accretion over decades of professional practices and standard operating procedures, does that suggest that health system reform supports the convergence thesis? Evans (2005) suggests that 'parallel evolution' might be a better way of explaining the evolution of health systems. He is particularly at pains to highlight the importance of the prevalent social values and power structures in a country since these determine the compromises among conflicting interests. He describes a common theme unfolding in each country, moving through two distinct phases. In the first phase, countries put in place some form of universal and comprehensive system of collective payment for health care, financed either through general taxation or compulsory social insurance. In the second phase, these same countries find themselves confronting the relentless pressure for cost escalation evident in all health care systems regardless of their method of financing. Trying to balance cost control while ensuring that the goals of access and public satisfaction, equity, effectiveness and efficiency are both protected and advanced is a tall order. It has proved an increasingly difficult task and in an effort to achieve it, governments have resorted to a range of supply-side reforms designed to manage rising demand on health care services. Rather than simply injecting more money into health services, governments have demanded that the way resources are spent be subject to closer scrutiny and reform. This has been an enduring theme of all governments and has most recently been expressed in *The National Health Service Five Year Forward View* (NHS England 2014).

While governments may be reluctant for good reason to alter the source of funding for health care, they are less protective of the way in which they are provided. In the case of the UK, or England to be more precise, the government has decided – in the absence, it must be said, of proper public debate – that as long as the funding of the NHS remains public and is allocated to each according to their needs, it does not matter who provides the services. What matters, according to the mantra, is what works. Therefore, to allow the private sector to provide services, either in place of, or in competition with, the NHS, is regarded as perfectly legitimate and a way of ensuring best value for money. The fact that there is no convincing or unequivocal evidence to substantiate such a policy has not deterred policy makers eager, if not doggedly determined, to prove the rightness of their (and especially perhaps their trusted advisers') policies. Indeed, what limited evidence there is suggests that reforms based on markets or market-like institutions and relying on competitive incentives to change provider behaviour have a particular tendency to generate inequities in access or regressive patterns of payment. In a market system, need is irrelevant. What counts is what pays best and maximises profit. For governments to be able to regulate such a market once established with the vigour and determination required flies in the face of all we know about market behaviour and the inability of governments to regulate effectively. Evans graphically captures the dilemma: 'Defeating this inherent tendency requires a strong and sophisticated regulatory environment, and structuring such an environment is like riding north on a southbound horse. There are powerful incentives for participants to erode or circumvent regulatory controls and move in the natural direction' (2005: 285–6).

In a painstaking analysis of over three decades of transforming government based on the mantra that by aping private business the public sector will get more efficient, two academics show that the running costs of central government have risen but without there being higher satisfaction levels (Hood and Dixon 2015). These rising costs, according to the study, can be put down to contracting out and outsourcing public services, which has resulted in a huge expansion of the consultancy sector.

The 'cult of managerialism'

If there has been a single prevailing feature characterising health system reforms in recent decades both in the UK and elsewhere, it is the 'cult of managerialism'. This has taken different forms and has, at times, emphasised bureaucratic aspects and at others market-type features in keeping with the global health system reform agenda and the centrality to this of market forces. But the reforms have in common a firm conviction that health systems require better management and that the weakness or absence of management accounts for avoidable inefficiencies and poor performance, and a tendency for professional monopolists exercising unbridled power to determine what happens in practice in respect of resource allocation and priority setting.

The commitment to stronger management has tended to follow 'Fordist' and/or 'post-Fordist' thinking as derived from Henry Ford (Harrison et al 1992). In turn, many of the principles underpinning this thinking have more than a passing resemblance to FW Taylor's school of 'scientific management'. At the core of these constructs is the notion that management needs to control the workforce by specifying in some detail what has to be done, how it is to be done, and in what quantity it is to be done. It is a mass production approach, oriented to efficiency and predictability and has been applied to health systems such as the British NHS. While retaining many of the Fordist features, post-Fordism seeks to fragment the organisation into its constituent parts, is more focused on results than with conforming to rules and procedures and seeks to be more consumer responsive. It shares much in common with new public management, which has had a major impact on the NHS and is considered later in the chapter.

Over the years, UK governments of all hues have experimented with various management fads and fashions ranging from consensus management, in vogue during the 1970s, to general management introduced in the 1980s. At times, a strong central pull has been evident; at other times, there have been moves to decentralise managerial authority and locate it with those providing frontline services. Over the past decade, both these countervailing forces have been in evidence, sometimes even simultaneously, but in the overall context of a government that is arguably the most managerial and technocratic of any in recent times. Not only do ministers speak the language of management and delivery, but they also act as the top management team steering the NHS despite the lack of any management experience. The problem is that new governments (as New Labour was in 1997), especially those that have been out of power for a long period and impatient to put their imprint on public services, believe that power resides with them and that they simply have to pull the levers to change direction without relying on, or trusting, others to do so. While there is some truth in this analysis of what has happened and why, it is far from being the whole picture, as Lipsky's (1980) study of street-level bureaucrats shows.

In time, all governments come to realise that the real world is considerably more messy and complex than they imagine and that, far from being in control, ministers and their advisers and officials are invariably the captives of the services they oversee (Mackenzie 1979). While they would probably protest that this is grossly unfair and point to the many improvements in the NHS since the investment of new resources, combined with the introduction and implementation of tough target and inspection regimes designed to reduce waiting times and improve access to care and its quality, these claimed successes have to be put in context and viewed with some caution. It may be true that there have indeed been real improvements, but holding targets and/or inspection largely responsible may be crediting them with more influence than is justified when the evidence is examined more closely. Conceivably, the improvements might have occurred anyway, in large part as a result of the injection of significant new funds following the Wanless review of challenges facing the NHS over the 20-year period up to 2022, but also because of sound management practices. Moreover, while aggressively imposed targets may have had some effect initially, it came at the price of clinical detachment and falling staff morale and, as noted earlier, evidence of widespread 'gaming'. A terror-by-target culture hardly seems conducive to winning the hearts and minds of those managing and providing services or to encouraging them to raise their game. Hence the government's change of tack with the change of prime minister in mid-2007, which has meant paying closer attention to how best to bring clinicians back into the fold, since they are seen as critical to the successful implementation of the reform agenda. The move away from central targets was taken a step further with the coalition government in 2010 when they were abolished – in theory if not in practice. The change was rather more presentational than substantive.

The managerial revolution in most health systems began in earnest in the 1980s and 1990s, although the British NHS was an early pioneer of management reforms. In 1974, the NHS underwent its first significant upheaval based on the work and concepts developed by a combination of international management consultants, McKinsey's, and Brunel University under Elliott Jacques and Ralph Rowbottom. The Brunel team invented a form of organisational analysis known as social analysis and it provided the theoretical and conceptual basis for the so-called official 'grey book' that described in some detail the architecture for the structure of the NHS as it emerged in the mid-1970s (Department of Health and Social Security 1972). For its part, McKinsey's work heralded the start of a long relationship with the NHS that continues to this day. Indeed, McKinsey's has been at the forefront of the market-style changes more recently introduced into the NHS. Its influence runs through these at every level but especially in its penetration of the central government department leading the changes, the Department of Health. We return to some of these developments in the next chapter.

New public management

The early managerial reforms were further developed in the 1980s and 1990s under the banner of 'new public management' (NPM), which lingers to this day. Some countries, including the UK and New Zealand, were regarded as the trailblazers of NPM, although its architect, Christopher Hood, saw it as a striking international trend in public administration observable from the mid-1970s onwards (Hood

1991). NPM has therefore become something of a global movement comprising a set of beliefs or an ideology as well as a set of doctrines governing public sector reform in services such as health systems, including the UK NHS (Dawson and Dargie 2002). Hood describes NPM as comprising seven doctrines, which he articulates as follows:

- a focus on hands-on and entrepreneurial management, as opposed to the traditional bureaucratic focus of the public administrator;
- explicit standards and measures of performance;
- an emphasis on output controls;
- the importance of disaggregation and decentralisation of public services;
- a shift to the promotion of competition in the provision of public services;
- a stress on private sector styles of management and their superiority;
- the promotion of discipline and parsimony in resource allocation.

Power has summarised the central ideas comprising NPM, suggesting that they were largely borrowed from private sector management thinking (Power 1997). Other critics have similarly seen NPM as a market-based ideology invading public sector organisations previously imbued with different values (Laughlin 1991; Rhodes 1996; Stewart 1998). Rhodes notes that NPM and entrepreneurial government 'share a concern with competition, markets, customers and outcomes' (1996: 655). Stewart believes that notwithstanding its slipperiness as a concept and its different emphasis in different countries, NPM is intent upon emulating in the public domain 'what is believed to be the practice of management in the private sector' (1998: 16). He continues:

> A rhetoric of an entrepreneurial approach has developed. There is the development of market mechanisms in place of hierarchy and an emphasis on the public as customer. Generally there is a tendency to simplify management tasks in the belief that clear targets and separation of roles can clarify responsibility and release management initiative.

> Simplification has been achieved by the separation of
> policy from implementation, the development of contracts,
> quasi-contracts or targets governing relationships, and their
> enforcement by performance management. This is believed
> to replicate an assumed clarity of tasks in the private sector.
> (Stewart 1998: 16)

Stewart offers a critique of these practices, believing that they 'are not
adequate as a basis for management in the public domain because they
are not based on the purposes, conditions and tasks of that domain'
(1998: 16). Moreover, NPM assumes that there is a model of private
sector management and that it can be applied to the public domain.
Stewart draws attention to the danger of an assumed private sector
model on the grounds that 'the distinctive features of the public domain
are neglected' (1998: 16).

Despite attempts to draw parallels between public and private
sector management, Whitley (1988) considers that the construction
of a general management science is as far away as ever. But Stewart's
criticism that NPM developed a rhetoric that identifies perceived
weaknesses in what may be termed traditional public administration
is important. As he suggests, charges of being 'over-bureaucratic',
'producer-dominated' and 'unresponsive' have been levelled at public
services such as the NHS in a way that caricatures a complex reality in
which there is a place for bureaucratic rules and procedures, and where
being unresponsive may have a place if the aim is to be impartial. Finally,
producer dominance may be a danger, but professional knowledge or
experience cannot be ignored altogether.

Some commentators have suggested that a formulation of NPM
based on mimicking the private sector in the public sector is in any
case too narrow and that the initial focus on the marketisation of
public services was broadened from 1997, under New Labour, towards
an emphasis on community governance (Osborne and McLaughlin
2002). Other commentators view NPM as a management hybrid,
fusing private and public sector management ideas, that still carries an
emphasis on core public service values (see, for example, discussion in

Chapter 1 of Ferlie et al 1996). While this may be so, the initial focus on NPM and the marketisation of public services remains valid, since a central feature of NPM is its assumption that public management is little different from private sector management and that it may have suffered from a perception that it is different, thereby failing to take full advantage of what are perceived to be the superior strengths of private management practices. This is another cleavage that remains unresolved and finds itself the source of constant attention in successive reform moves. However, as Hood and others, such as Ferlie et al (1996), agree, NPM is of much greater significance than the usual fad or fashion.

What is also remarkable and not in dispute is, as Marmor (2004) noted, how widely and rapidly these ideas spread throughout governments and public services such as the NHS. This is why the notion of NPM as a movement has a particular resonance. At its core was the idea that public services were inefficient, unresponsive to user preferences and often ineffective. They were run, it was alleged, more for the convenience of providers, principally clinicians, than for those who depended on them. High cost went hand in hand with poor performance. As a result of this critique, the ground was prepared for major reform that sought to mimic in the public sector the best of business or private sector management practices. To this day, the NHS has been subjected to more of this type of thinking than any other public service. It was, as Ferlie et al observe, 'an early and rapid mover in this field' (1996: 27), adopting general management in the early 1980s and quasi-market principles in the late 1980s/early 1990s. In fact, as noted above, elements of NPM thinking in the NHS can be traced back to its first major reorganisation in 1974. Of course, there were strict limits on how far market-style thinking could be applied to a public service such as health care, so the term 'quasi-market' was used. In particular, the NHS had a capped budget determined annually by government. And, second, a true market with winners and losers was not seen to be viable or politically acceptable in the NHS.

The UK NHS was not the only health system active in reforming its health care structures. Another pioneer was New Zealand, where market reforms proved even more radical and went further than anything evident elsewhere. In fact, such zeal for market reforms, which waned during the mid- and late 1990s, did not become evident again until around 2003 in the UK with the government's latest set of changes. This is despite the perception in New Zealand that its reforms had gone too far, and achieved only negligible success.

In response to criticisms that NPM reforms resulted in fragmentation and inappropriate competition, a new generation of reforms appeared with labels such as 'joined-up government' (JUG) and 'whole of government' (Christensen and Laegreid 2007). These concepts sought to apply a more holistic strategy using insights from the other social sciences in place of an almost exclusive reliance on economics and the narrow, reductionist, efficiency focus of NPM to which an economics perspective gave credence (Hunter 2006a). But they were hardly new: the issue of coordination has been of long-standing concern in government and in the context of 'wicked issues' that straddle the boundaries of public sector organisations, administrative levels and policy areas. In contrast to first-generation NPM reforms, JUG was presented as an antidote to 'departmentalism' and 'vertical silos'. NPM reforms from the 1980s and 1990s focused on performance management, meeting targets aimed at single-purpose organisations, and on vertical coordination. The result may have been too much fragmentation and an absence of cooperation and coordination, deficits for which Rhodes (1996) holds NPM responsible because of an absence of the trust necessary to manage inter-organisational networks and to reach what Strauss et al (1964) term 'a negotiated order'.

Reflecting on the period of health system reform commencing in the mid-1970s gives rise to a number of questions. Two in particular stand out. First, what fuelled the health system reform movement at this time and subsequently as it gathered pace through successive decades? And, second, why the focus on management and on seeing managers as effectively a means of wresting power from doctors in order better to align health system goals with those of policy makers and patients? The answers may lie in the repositioning of New Labour's health system reform strategy starting in the late 1990s and continuing to the present day. Despite the coalition government's reform strategy being presented as a way of freeing up clinicians, notably GPs, to make decisions in the best interests of their patients, the reality has proved rather different. We return to this conundrum in the next chapter.

The NHS chief executive in England, Simon Stevens, who became one of the most influential advisers in the Blair government in Britain in his capacity first as adviser to two secretaries of state for health before being elevated to become the prime minister's health adviser, suggested that the reform strategies adopted by New Labour had their origins in a perception that the NHS could not survive without an injection of significant resources. Otherwise, the gap between the NHS's performance and growing public expectations would widen and those who could afford to would exit from the NHS, resulting in it becoming a residualist safety net (Stevens 2004). But, crucially, it was also accepted that the extra investment would need to deliver more consumer-responsive health care and that serious management weaknesses remained despite several earlier reforms and restructuring. It was believed that the history of NHS reform since the mid-1970s had been marked by a continuing failure to manage clinical work effectively (Harrison et al 1992). As a result, in the words of a former Conservative health minister, Patrick Jenkin, the NHS was 'overadministered and undermanaged'. So, without the combination of additional investment and reform, taxpayers would come to regard the NHS model as *the* problem rather than underfunding or poor political stewardship. Consequently, having committed themselves to several years of significant growth in NHS spending that, as intended, would bring the NHS closer to the European average in terms of spending on health, policy makers' attention switched to supply-side changes in order to secure a better return on their investment. The focus shifted to expanding output, improving quality and increasing responsiveness while avoiding cost inflation. Such an agenda continued under the coalition government, although its complex, and many would argue unnecessary, NHS structural changes dominated its term of office between 2010 and 2015.

Grappling with such issues gave rise to three waves of health reform soon after New Labour's arrival in office in May 1997 and also informed the coalition government's 'big bang' changes announced in July 2010, which in various ways sought to address the 'management problem' in the NHS. These are the subject of Chapter Four, which is concerned with models of health system reform. Looking back at the various waves of health system reform in the UK over the past 30 years or so, it is possible to pick out a number of recurring, and often overlapping, themes and issues that have been the subject of endless debate, among them the following:

- public versus private approaches to the provision of health care;
- the changing relationship between clinicians and managers;
- the oscillation from centralisation to decentralisation;
- command and control versus markets;
- attempts to strengthen the public and patient voice;
- the tension between a focus on downstream acute health care, and upstream public health and health prevention.

Virtually all health care reforms have wrestled in various ways with all, or some combination of, these issues in order to arrive at a different set of dynamics and incentives. But, for the most part, none of them is resolved in any final or lasting sense; they remain in constant tension with the dialectic between them being played out, or replayed, in each successive wave of reform. The next chapter provides some illustrations of this dilemma. But we are nevertheless left with the problem of management and whether the expectations of it are too high and unrealistic. Marmor suggests that managerial fads give the lie to believing 'that there is some one right way, some panacea, for rationalising the delivery of decent, affordable medical care' (2004: 22). In fact, he contends, 'management is not a solution to seemingly intractable stresses. Rather, it is a means of coping with and sometimes improving only marginally tractable situations' (Marmor 2004: 23). Despite the history of the NHS being littered with the debris of failed managerial fads that offer oversimplified answers to complex problems, it is a lesson that policy makers have yet to learn. Humility has never been uppermost in their framework of competencies; nor has any appreciation of history.

Back to the future?

The use of history in health policy making in the UK has been explored by Virginia Berridge (2007). Drawing on her own policy experience and interviews she conducted with key informants involved in the policy process, she found that historical analysis has no formal role in policy, although it was nonetheless being used in an ad hoc way, particularly in justifying the adoption of a political line that might appear controversial such as equating NHS foundation trusts (hospitals that remained part of the NHS family and accountable to the secretary of state for health but were granted a degree of freedom from central control, having earned their autonomy through improvements in the quality of care provided) with the mutual tradition (Berridge 2007). The use of history, like other disciplines such as political science or organisation behaviour, is linked to a more general issue about the sources of advice and evidence available within government. It seems that of the various sources of information used by policy makers, special advisers come top of the list followed by 'experts', think tanks, lobbyists, pressure groups, professional associations, the media and finally constituents and users. Academics are not 'on the radar', although it is possible to identify a few who have been influential such as Julian Le Grand, mentioned earlier. However, none has been an historian. Therefore, where history has been invoked, historians have rarely been involved in the process. And yet, a failure to learn from past experience is possibly one of the main reasons for organisational failure in health. Certainly, the history of NHS reorganisations would counsel caution in respect of the government's fixation on organisational restructuring as an instrument of bringing about real and lasting change.

The various NHS reforms, especially those occurring from the late 1980s onwards, are often regarded as examples of novelty, progressive thinking and modernity. But when analysed more closely there is very little that is actually new about them. Hence Metcalfe and Richards' comment that NPM succeeded only in dragging Britain 'kicking and screaming back into the 1950s' (quoted in Rhodes 1996: 663). As far as the NHS reforms are concerned, for the most part there are strong parallels with the pre-1948 arrangements for the organisation and delivery of health care. As Mohan (2002) observes, public–private partnerships are heralded as new delivery vehicles but in the case of hospital provision they represent a reversion to the 1930s and 1940s. More recently, the enthusiasm for social enterprises in the running of health and social care has strong echoes of the voluntary hospital system that preceded the NHS (Mohan 2003). Then, there was a diverse, plural mixed economy of care with a strong emphasis on local ownership and variation, and on being attentive to individual preferences. In the end, the degree of variation that ensued was regarded as intolerable and the birth of the NHS was the response. Some 67 years later, the government is putting in place changes that surely threaten to create a similar set of pressures. As Mohan puts it:

> Like the Ministry of Health in the 1930s, the government seems willing to accept a degree of localism and variability in order to continue to secure continual support for the NHS. If the implication of the current trajectory of policy is that the NHS will become a much more diverse collection of services than in its history to date, the issue then will become the degree of inequity that is tolerable. (Mohan 2002: 223)

Had the lessons from history been learned, it is conceivable that developments such as foundation hospital trusts and their governance structures, and the much-heralded return to mutualism, might have taken a different turn or at least been undertaken with greater awareness of the historical record (Gorsky 2006). It is also inconceivable that the coalition government's changes would have succeeded in getting onto the statute book. Yet they did, despite widespread opposition from NHS staff and the public – at least those members of it who understood the complex and rather technical changes proposed.

As Gauld (2001) observes in regard to market-style reforms in New Zealand, it is doubtful that these reflect the real world of public policy since they have been pursued in response to flawed supporting assumptions. Echoing Stewart's analysis of the limitations of NPM thinking noted earlier, he draws attention to the 'fundamental differences' between private sector markets and the so-called 'market' for public goods that makes the marketisation of public services problematic. The solution to imperfect markets in areas such as health and health care is invariably some form of government involvement, usually in one of three forms, or a mix of these: regulating private markets; monitoring and controlling the flow of resources to ensure that people receive appropriate care and do so equitably; or providing the services in their entirety. In practice, policy makers in different health systems pursue a mix of these options since none on its own has proved entirely satisfactory. Indeed, as is often said, there is no such thing as a perfect health system, merely less imperfection; therefore governments are always negotiating and renegotiating the optimum mix of policy instruments to achieve their desired ends. Health system reform resembles a swinging pendulum that oscillates between extremes. For example, sometimes the swing is towards centralisation and at other times towards decentralisation (as is evident, for example, in the government's Northern Powerhouse initiative aimed at devolving powers and resources, including control over the NHS, to local government in the North and elsewhere, starting with Greater Manchester [Association of Greater Manchester Authority et al 2015]). And sometimes it is towards markets and competition, while at other times it is towards direct provision and collaboration. As we have seen, often fashion dictates the swing of the pendulum in a particular direction. But it can also be affected by policy makers being persuaded by a particular ideological direction that may itself have been exported from, or have its origins in, another country and context.

The question to be asked, surely, is at what point in the future will something not so dissimilar to the NHS that in its present form is, in the view of some observers, being 'hollowed out' while retaining the brand, be given a makeover and regarded as modern and progressive? It seems that public sector reform has become more like the fashion industry than may be desirable or comfortable to contemplate. However, history rarely repeats itself exactly and it may be that the health system in England (health services elsewhere in the UK so far seem less inclined to follow the English lead) begins to resemble something more akin to a European system in respect of its complexity, plurality and diversity. The NHS brand may then be up for sale.

Conclusion

The predominant approach to NHS reform in the UK has been twofold: a focus on centralised targets and inspection, together with a growing commercialisation of health care services. The fact that these two approaches are in potential conflict with each other has only served to create what Lawson calls 'a cocktail of fears about health inequalities as well as a host of unintended consequences and inefficiencies. It has led to the alienation of staff and widespread uncertainty among the public' (2007: 4).

The honeymoon enjoyed by the New Labour government in Britain when first elected in 1997, and the enormous goodwill shown towards it, was well and truly over by 2002. That goodwill remains in short supply and was not restored when the coalition government entered office in 2010. Few observers have dissented from the government's diagnosis of the problems or challenges facing the NHS. But it is elements of the prescription for change, notably a belief that the only way to bring about lasting change is to open up health services to market-style competition and choice, and the manner in which the government has chosen to prosecute the change agenda, that have given rise to growing concerns among NHS staff and sections of the public. Few of these changes have been actively discussed with, or informed by, key stakeholders within the NHS and none has been publicly debated. The government has proceeded on the basis that it knows best and that to allow clinicians and others to influence the reform agenda would risk diluting or distorting it and losing its radical edge. Hence, regardless of what ministers may say to the contrary, their determination to micro-manage the changes from the centre and to keep close control of their progress and impact remains undiminished. In contrast to the management rhetoric at the time, where it was suggested by writers such as Osborne and Gaebler (1993) that governments should steer more and row less, the government not only sees its role as one of steering but of rowing vigorously, too.

Underlying successive governments' approach is a deep-seated lack of trust that managers can achieve its reforms despite the fact that managers have been among its chief beneficiaries. The entire thrust of NPM appears to be based on mistrust rather than trust. Rather, it is central government that will decide when to grant autonomy (as captured in the idea of 'earned autonomy') and when to withhold it. The effect has been to politicise yet further the management of the NHS, with managers ever more inclined to look upwards to ministers rather than downwards into their organisations, and outwards to their local communities. Such an orientation has arguably bred a dependency culture and what can best be described as a type of managerial infantilism that can only lead to weak management of the very kind the government ostensibly wishes to remove. It is another paradox and a further example of the government's actions intended to achieve one outcome actually resulting in a quite different one. The government's abiding faith in a particular type of crude and largely discredited managerialism, which has accompanied its three phases of reform, is explored further in Chapter Four. Before then, we turn to the issue of health and wellbeing and the NHS's part in this, which is in fact rather limited given the other factors and pressures shaping people's health. But that may be about to change.

THREE

Moving upstream: the dilemma of securing health in health policy

Introduction

One of the most protracted and impassioned debates in health policy concerns the imbalance between the attention and resources devoted to health care as distinct from health. Virtually all the attention from policy makers, professionals, public and media, together with the bulk of resources available, are focused on ill-health, sickness and disease. It is a curious irony that few health systems pay much attention to health, focusing instead on ill-health and disease. They are diagnose-and-treat systems rather than systems designed to predict and prevent, and operate in such a fashion even when making a pretence of putting health before health care. A good example of this tendency can be found in a speech delivered by a former British health secretary, Alan Milburn. The lecture was given in 2002, two years after Milburn launched Labour's 10-Year Plan for Health and Care, which, in contrast to the message delivered in his lecture, focused almost exclusively on health care services. His lecture was an impassioned plea for putting health before health care: 'The health debate in our country has for too long been focused on the state of the nation's health service and not enough on the state of the nation's health'. He continued: 'The time has now come to put renewed emphasis on prevention as well as treatment…. It is time for a sea change in attitudes' (Milburn 2002: 1). But arguably, the issue is not a lack of strategies or policies. As Derek Wanless, special adviser to Brown and Blair on the future challenges facing the NHS up to 2022, wryly commented, 'what is striking is that there has been so much written often covering similar ground and apparently sound, setting out the well-known major determinants of health, but rigorous implementation of identified solutions has often been sadly lacking' (Wanless 2004: 3). Given the evidence of little change on the ground, what is needed, he argues, 'is delivery and implementation, not further discussion' (Wanless 2004: 183).

Over the past 14 years or so since Wanless produced his two reports on the state of the nation's health setting out recommendations that the then Labour government endorsed, little has changed. If anything, the position in regard to lifestyle-related illnesses has deteriorated, while the gap between the better off and worse off has increased (National Audit Office 2010) as have levels of health inequality between the North and South of the country (Whitehead 2014). And this is on top of the independent review of health inequalities post-2010 commissioned by the last Labour government and conducted by Michael Marmot (Marmot 2010). The coalition government from 2010–15 presided over the biggest NHS and public health reorganisation since 1974 and the accompanying upheaval proved distracting for those seeking to improve health and wellbeing. Moreover, the government adopted tough fiscal measures to reduce the deficit and control public spending. Yet, as Sen (2015) and other distinguished economists have argued, austerity measures were a political choice and not required to rescue the economy after the financial collapse in 2008. Indeed, such measures have slowed growth and recovery. They have also hit public sector services and employees hardest of all, especially those run and employed by local government. Following the UK general election in May 2015 and the election of a Conservative government with a slim overall majority, further deep cuts are to be imposed and for reasons which have little to do with sound economic management but everything to do with political positioning and neoliberal ideology.

During Labour's first term in office (1997–2001), there was an almost palpable belief and confidence in the ability of government to bring about real change in health, and not only health care, and also to make significant inroads into widening health inequalities. There was an enthusiasm to embrace new and innovative solutions and to learn from their experience. Enlightened and innovative government action, it was believed, could make a real difference to the lives of individuals and to impoverished communities. But, as noted above, by 2000 the government's focus had shifted from health back to health care and issues such as waiting lists and times, access to beds and balancing the books consumed its attention. In contrast to England, Wales and Scotland sought to give a higher priority to health improvement and narrowing the health gap (Smith et al 2008). There was a desire in both countries to see health improvement as part of a broader social justice agenda. And to an extent this focus on health and wellbeing in their widest sense remains a distinguishing feature of the devolved governance arrangements in the UK (Timmins 2013).

Another development took place, too, with implications for public health policy that persist to this day, namely, the growing embrace of market-style thinking and neoliberal principles in England from around 2002 onwards, stressing individual lifestyle issues and downplaying the socioeconomic structural determinants of health and the role of government in tackling them (Hunter 2005). Such a shift was manifest in the second English public health White Paper, *Choosing Health*, published in 2004 (Secretary of State for Health 2004). It received further endorsement in July 2006 in a major speech on public health delivered by the then prime minister, Tony Blair, in which he referred to the new challenges facing society whether from smoking, poor diet, alcohol misuse or sexual behaviour. He claimed that 'our public health problems are not, strictly speaking, public health questions at all. They are questions of individual lifestyle' (Blair 2006). Such a view marked a decisive shift in thinking and could be contrasted with the focus on social determinants underpinning earlier health policy. Some years on the government's stance remained confused. For instance, in his first major speech as health secretary, Alan Johnson argued for stronger government intervention to tackle unhealthy lifestyles and at the same time stressed the limits to government action. He stated: 'government simply can't afford to be passive observers of unhealthy lifestyles', only intervening once diseases have become manifest (Johnson 2007). He also believed that 'the public are now less concerned about a nanny state than they are about a neglectful state'. But in another sentence he said it is 'down to personal responsibility', thereby implying that government can educate, advise and inform but not intervene to create circumstances and/or environments in which people might be able to lead healthier lives. Yet, in respect of many contemporary public health problems, such as obesity, the need is for action at a societal as well as at an individual level. Such confusion continued to permeate health policy when the coalition government emerged after the 2010 election and continues to do so under the Conservative government elected in May 2015, as we shall see later in this chapter.

There is some truth in the claim that the Labour government was the first in a generation to recognise health inequalities as a priority and it did attempt to face up to it. To be fair, there were some positive gains and achievements, especially in terms of tackling child poverty and introducing the minimum wage and tax credits to alleviate poverty among working families. Action on child poverty succeeded in arresting and reversing the rising long-term trend. Whereas in 1997 there were 3.4 million children in poverty – one in three children – by 2005/06 there were 600,000 fewer children in relative low-income households than in 1998/99 (Department of Health 2008a). Tax credit measures announced in the 2007 budget would lift a further 300,000 children out of poverty from April 2008. In terms of the population as a whole and in absolute terms, health was getting better, with life expectancy for all social groups going up and infant mortality figures going down.

But these modest gains notwithstanding, critics argued that the Labour government failed to do enough either in terms of publicly confronting the problem of poverty and health inequalities or in its policies, and that for all the successes in some areas, the evidence overall pointed to a worsening position in respect of health inequality as measured by life expectancy and infant mortality. Indeed the government's own evidence bore this out as published in a series of status reports by the Department of Health (Department of Health 2008a). This showed that the life expectancy gap between men living in the poorest areas of England and the average male was 2% wider than it was in the preceding 10 years.

The period of the coalition government from 2010 to 2015 witnessed a reversal of the modest gains under Labour and a widening of health inequalities (Schrecker and Bambra 2015). The trends seem destined to worsen further under the Conservative government elected in May 2015, given its determination to stick to its austerity policy and to go further in making public spending cuts. Indeed, one of the Chancellor's first acts was to announce an emergency budget in which he cut £200 million from the public health budget that will directly affect local government and represents a 7% reduction in its total public health spend.

With significant inequalities in wealth and health remaining, this could hardly be said to amount to an impressive track record of achievement, especially if, as many believe, income inequality does matter – not the absolute levels of income but the extent of the income gap between social groups (Wilkinson 2005; Wilkinson and Pickett 2009).

This was the situation that the coalition government inherited in 2010. Like its predecessors, the government also focused heavily on the NHS and health care services, although it did acknowledge the importance of public health. Indeed, it took the view that since tackling the social determinants of health was more suited to local government than the NHS, it made more sense for public health to return there. Prior to the 1974 NHS reorganisation, public health had been the responsibility of local government and many regretted its shift to the NHS (Hunter et al 2010). Even critics of the changes to the NHS welcomed the coalition government's public health changes, although some, mainly public health clinicians, saw the move as reckless and undesirable (McKee et al 2011).

Putting health before health care has defeated successive governments that have ultimately lacked the political will to tackle the vested interests contributing to ill-health. The public health White Paper published in November 2010 (Secretary of State for Health 2010a), apart from moving public health responsibilities from the NHS to local authorities, announced for the first time the ring-fencing of the public health budget estimated at over £4 billion. The move to local government was defended on the grounds that it is better placed than the NHS to address the social determinants of health and engage local people in the broader health improvement agenda. Local government, it was claimed, possesses many of the levers for promoting wellbeing and shaping local communities in a healthy direction. Tackling health inequalities was an area where local government had considerable experience and was able to take action in regard to housing, economic and environmental regeneration, education, fire and road safety and so on.

The NHS reforms introduced in 2013 are considered in the next chapter but the view held by the coalition government was that liberating the NHS from excessive central control would fundamentally change the role of the Department of Health and make it more strategic, focused 'on improving public health, tackling health inequalities' (Secretary of State for Health 2010b). Central public health functions were to become the responsibility of a new arm's length agency, Public Health England.

The public health reforms were broadly welcomed, especially by those who wished to see a more social model of health prevail in place of a biomedical model focused on ill-health and disease. But critics wondered how far devolving responsibility for public health to local government would put at risk a national approach to improving health and wellbeing and tackling inequalities. Since many of the forces leading to poor health were the responsibility of national governments, how far local authorities could address these on their own was a key concern. There were also concerns about how localist the changes in fact were, with at least one critic alleging that while the language and rhetoric of the White Paper were localist, its proposals were prescriptive and top-down when it came to the national outcomes framework, proposals for how health and wellbeing boards should function and so on (Coppard 2010). The fear was that local priorities would be undermined or overridden by national imperatives. Even the ring-fenced budget was criticised for acting as a barrier to adopting a whole-systems approach and reducing the freedom of local authorities to decide how best to utilise available funds.

Despite an incoming administration once again expressing a commitment to tackling the wider determinants of health and reducing health inequalities in society, the coalition government failed to make much headway. Like its predecessors, it had no desire to do battle with those vested interests in the food and drink sector. It was content to introduce a system of responsibility deals, whereby all the key interests would come together and reach voluntary agreements on the levels of sugar and salt in food. The government maintained that if progress were not fast enough, it would legislate for reductions, but the emphasis was firmly on not going down this route. Critics of the policy argue that the government was determined to appease corporate interests, many of which donated sums to the Conservative Party and lobbied heavily to influence policy. On alcohol minimum unit pricing there was also disappointment following a promising start with the prime minister calling for action. In the end, while Scotland did act (although the proposals are subject to legal challenge in the European courts and have yet to be implemented), England chose not to. Only in regard to smoking cessation and the introduction of plain packaging has there been modest progress, although it took most of the coalition government's five-year term of office, with lengthy periods of foot dragging and delay while the evidence base was re-reviewed, to achieve this.

Overall, then, by 2015 and despite public health having been high on the policy agenda since the Labour government entered office in 1997, successive governments have failed to make significant headway in putting health before health care. Indeed, in some respects we may be losing ground. While returning public health to local government in England has much to commend it for reasons already given, it has occurred at a time when local government has been subjected to severe public spending cuts that are seriously affecting its capacity to function effectively. The Chancellor's unexpected announcement in June to reduce public health funding by £200 million hardly seemed to be in keeping with the call in *The National Health Service Five Year Forward View* for 'a radical upgrade in prevention and public health' (NHS England 2014: 3). This strategy document noted that Wanless's warning,

THE HEALTH DEBATE [SECOND EDITION]

issued back in 2002, that unless prevention was taken seriously we would be faced with a sharply rising burden of preventable illness 'has not been heeded – and the NHS is on the hook for the consequences' (NHS England 2014: 3). It does seem that governments struggle to adopt a systems-wide perspective when it comes to health and health care, failing to see the connections between the different parts of the system. Yet, it is precisely transformational change along these lines to enhance population health that is being called for by developed health systems (Halfon et al 2014).

Which factors account for the persistence of a central dilemma in health policy whereby governments of all persuasions find it difficult to provide a robust and sustainable lead on public health issues, opting in the end to leave it to individuals to make up their own minds? The next sections explore the dilemma further.

Health care before health

While only about 10% of people are treated in hospital, some 90% of resources allocated to health services are devoted to acute care in hospital. In contrast, only around 4% of health resources are allocated to health prevention measures. To reinforce the point, as one commentator shrewdly observed, how often do politicians when they stand up at party political conferences or similar events talk about health? Even when they invoke the term, what they invariably mean, and go on to eulogise over, is hospitals, beds and buildings, and the numbers of doctors and nurses employed. Of course, politicians cannot be entirely blamed for adopting such a narrow focus. Much of the media and the public ascribes to a similarly narrow view of health and what contributes to it, as, indeed, do many of those working in the NHS. If politicians rarely put public health first, they are closely followed by health care managers and clinicians.

An exception to the rule is the NHS chief executive, Simon Stevens, who was appointed in April 2014. Unusually for a health care manager, he takes every opportunity publicly to speak about the importance of public health and in *The National Health Service Five Year Forward*

View, investment in public health is given a high priority as one of the measures to ensure the sustainability of a publicly funded health care system (NHS England 2014). But shifting the focus is hard, even when the evidence in an area such as obesity points to the need for urgent action by government and others. Political and managerial careers are shaped by tangible achievements and while good health is largely invisible, the means by which ill-health and disease are tackled are all too visible and hold a strong emotional appeal. On the assumption that politicians and senior managers should on occasion provide leadership rather than merely follow public opinion, there exists a major imbalance in the discourse of health policy.

Whatever the reason for the imbalance, it is important to remind ourselves of its persistence. The phenomenon is neither new nor confined to particular countries or their health systems. Health systems, as we have noted, in their broadest sense are about promoting and producing health. The precise contribution of health services in the pursuit of health is a hotly contested issue in health policy, with some observers claiming that the services have little to contribute to improved health while others argue the opposite. The truth, as ever, probably lies somewhere in between. Health services do contribute to quality of life, particularly in respect of people suffering from a chronic illness. It is also a contributor to the decline of avoidable mortality among infants and in deaths among middle-aged and older people (Nolte and McKee 2004). But though it may be conceded that health services probably contribute more to promoting and maintaining health than was previously thought, there remain powerful and persuasive arguments about whether the balance is right between investing in the prevention of ill-health or in its treatment, and in determining whose responsibility it is. As the Nuffield Council on Bioethics states in its important report on public health, many of the major advances in population health have been the result of non-medical developments (Nuffield Council on Bioethics 2007). These include advances in housing, drainage and sanitation. Medical advances, notably immunisation and vaccination programmes, have played their part, too.

Central to the dilemma of achieving an optimal balance between promoting better health and alleviating ill-health is the degree to which promoting health is regarded as an issue governed by individual lifestyle or one where structural determinants have the greater leverage on health status. Whichever driver for better health is regarded as more important will determine the requisite policy response. Of course, it may be that a combination of policies aimed at changing both individual lifestyle and structural determinants is favoured, but even so, it will still be necessary to determine where the balance should lie in terms of effort, resource and action. When it comes to deciding who is responsible for public health, in most countries the lead role for promoting health and preventing ill-health has been accorded to the health service. Other options are possible. For example, as noted earlier, in the UK prior to 1974, principal responsibility for public health lay with local government. Each local authority had a Medical Officer of Health, whose job it was to monitor the health of the population. And in 2013, in England, the lead for public health reverted to local government, with Directors of Public Health and their teams transferring from the NHS. Although joint posts between local government and the NHS had existed for a number of years before then, the public health function was seen to lie primarily with the NHS. This is no longer the case.

It is an interesting time for health policy in Europe and beyond. There is a growing recognition that simply pouring resources into health care services, especially those centred on acute hospital care, cannot be equated with good health. Indeed, such services will before long become unaffordable and unsustainable in terms of their public funding from social insurance or taxation unless efforts are made to manage demand and move health policy in a different direction. The so-called 'diseases of comfort' – the primary cause of death in the 21st century and the next – demand a different approach. It is one that requires government action and is not simply based on blaming individuals for their unhealthy lifestyles and relying on behaviour change to address the problem (Choi et al 2005; Kawachi 2007).

Policy makers face a variety of policy dilemmas arising from diseases of comfort. These do not lie principally in a lack of understanding. There is ample research and analysis testifying to the high levels of poor health evident in our societies and the extent of a widening health gap between social groups (see, for example, Mackenbach 2005). There is also a sizeable body of evidence on what needs to be done about these failings, although there remain research gaps in our knowledge of which interventions work and are most effective. Among the chief impediments to securing sustainable change is the absence of effective governance arrangements, coupled with the absence of a sustained political will to effect change that may take years to show results. Whether it is the obesity pandemic, growing alcohol misuse or the widening health gap between rich and poor, society's efforts to deal with such complex public policy challenges appear weak and inadequate. Too much emphasis is placed on changing individuals' behaviour and on repairing the damage once it has occurred rather than on preventing it in the first place. In the jargon, the focus is on downstream measures that deal with symptoms instead of upstream intervention that tackles the root causes of modern health problems.

As noted above, there is also a tendency to focus too narrowly on people's health problems and deficits that require professional expertise for their resolution rather than turning this on its head and looking at which factors keep people healthy and at the resources they possess that might be developed in a creative and positive manner to improve health. In short, we remain wedded to a biomedical model of health rather than a social ecological model. Moreover, we – or rather politicians – assume that all technological and scientific change is progressive and modern and is to be enthusiastically embraced even when such change may be to the detriment of our health.

What is meant by 'diseases of comfort'? By this term is meant principally those chronic diseases caused by obesity and physical inactivity. They underlie the three public health questions dominating policy discussion in many countries and their health systems:

- what is really driving the global chronic disease epidemic?
- why are demands on health care rising, putting growing pressure on health care expenditure?
- what has to happen to stem the rising tide of obesity and physical inactivity?

Running through each of these questions is the role of human progress and civilisation as contributing factors to the chronic disease epidemic. One view, which as noted above tends to be favoured by politicians, suggests that human history is a record of continuous progress towards perfection. An alternative view, and reading of history, is that the search for perfection and the assumption of 'progress' that accompanies it is misplaced. Certain inventions and technological and other changes neither improve on the present nor represent progress. While we celebrate scientific knowledge alongside economic growth and productivity, we should be aware of their impact on the poor, on work–life balance, on stress levels in the workforce and on lifestyles – effects such as physical inactivity, poor diet, smoking and excessive alcohol consumption – that could be, and indeed are, damaging to health. The modern myth is that science enables humanity to take charge of its collective destiny. But, as John Gray, professor of European Thought at the London School of Economics, has argued, 'in truth there are only humans using the growing knowledge given them by science to pursue their conflicting ends' (Gray 2003: 4).

We therefore urgently need a new paradigm to enable us to confront the diseases of comfort and the failings of our health care systems to tackle these as presently conceived and configured. Advocates of public health believe that unless we make the step change necessary to combat anti-health forces wherever these occur, public health will continue both to collude with, and remain eclipsed by, acute health care services and all the issues accompanying this that dominate the attention of policy makers, such as waiting lists and access to hospital beds. At the same time, our societies will become sicker rather than healthier. We (and policy makers) have a choice. We can go the way of the US, the country that spends most on its health care but has among the poorest outcomes for its population. Or we can look to Japan, Cuba and some Scandinavian countries, all of which, in their different ways, recognise the importance of a healthy society for a healthy economy and have the outcomes to support this. In the case of Japan and Cuba, it must be said, this is achieved with significantly lower per capita health care expenditure.

Achieving good health and wellbeing is a multifaceted and complex matter. For example, the Foresight report on obesity, prepared by the office of the government chief scientist in the UK, concludes that the country is on course for 60% of adult men, 50% of adult women and about 25% of all children under 16 becoming obese by 2050 (Butland et al 2007). Because the causes of obesity are extremely complex, encompassing biology and behaviour, the report says the responsibility for such a state of affairs cannot be pinned on individuals and their lifestyles. It asserts that we have created an obesogenic environment (or what some have termed a 'globesogenic' problem since it is of global dimensions) that requires action from government and communities at various levels. 'A bold whole system approach is critical' and will require 'a broad set of integrated policies including both population and targeted measures and must necessarily include action not only by government ... but also action by industry, communities, families and society as a whole' (Butland et al 2007: Summary of key messages). The Foresight team notes that obesity has much in common with other public health challenges or what have been termed 'wicked issues' (Hunter, Marks and Smith 2010).

Since the landmark Foresight report, insufficient action has been taken in terms of public policy to meet the challenge. At best, governments remain content to nudge people towards healthier behaviour through such means as including calorie counts on menus, or reducing portion sizes or the number of holes in salt cellars. This is despite evidence that demonstrates that shove, through taxation and/or regulation, rather than nudge policies alone are far more effective. The lack of action at scale means that the obesity crisis has worsened. It is now a critical global issue. According to the McKinsey Global Institute, 'more than 2.1 billion people – close to 30 percent of the global population – today are overweight or obese' (Dobbs et al 2014: 1). In tackling the problem, and echoing the Foresight report from seven years earlier, it is widely acknowledged that no single intervention will have sufficient impact to reverse obesity. Accepting the limits of personal actions, the McKinsey report states that while education and personal responsibility are important in reducing obesity, 'they are not enough on their own', and need to be accompanied by changes in the environment and societal norms. There is no shortage of analysis of the problem or even of what needs to be done. What is missing is the political will to act, a key ingredient that is missing from the McKinsey report. Yet such will is required if the action NHS England calls for is to be implemented. It will support 'hard-hitting and broad-based national action' that goes beyond individual behaviour change to include 'wider changes to distribution, marketing, pricing, and product formulation'. More recently Public Health England has entered the debate on obesity with a hard-hitting evidence-based review on the need to control the excess consumption of sugar (Tedstone et al 2015). The report opens with the stark statement: 'We are eating too much sugar and it is bad for our health' (p 5). Among its proposed eight key actions, most of which require government-led action, is a controversial recommendation for a 10-20% tax on sugary soft drinks. Although backed by food campaigner and celebrity chef, Jamie Oliver, and having public support according to some polls, such a tax has been rejected by the prime minister, David Cameron. Some campaigners favour reformulation of food to reduce the amount of sugar as a higher priority. It remains to be seen just how far the government is willing to take action that goes beyond raising awareness of concerns around excess sugar consumption when it publishes its whole of government child obesity strategy in early 2016. Whether the government's responsibility deal is sufficient to achieve these changes is arguable. Most public health advocates fear it is not, given the limited progress so far, and the evidence that such voluntary agreements are effective is not encouraging (Bryden et al 2013).

We also know that health and happiness are linked. As the work of economist Richard Layard (2005) and others shows, health and happiness go together and both result in more productive and viable communities. Yet, despite the achievement of successful and growing economies, it does not appear that these axiomatically lead to more contented, happier societies. Indeed, the evidence would suggest otherwise, especially in regard to the rising number of people suffering from mild mental illness. This phenomenon, according to the psychologist Oliver James (2007), is a consequence of a modern affliction he terms 'Affluenza', another disease of comfort. Of course, some people thrive in the new flexible economy and feel empowered by it, so it may not all be bad for our health, but, as the sociologist Richard Sennett's work amply shows, whole groups in society are increasingly marginalised or living lives that are sub-optimal and well below their potential resulting in a corrosion of character (Sennett 1999 and 2006).

The problem: the dominance of the medical model

So there is a dilemma facing health policy and it is essentially a political one involving the unequal distribution of power vested in certain interests and professional groups, which can lead to poor physical and mental health and a less productive and happy workforce. Paradoxically, although the population is living longer and is healthier overall than at any time in human history, it also contains within it the seeds of its own destruction, as evident in problems such as obesity – regarded as the new epidemic. A former Chief Medical Officer for England suggested that as a result of the rise of non-communicable diseases, we are creating a generation of children who will be outlived by their parents (Department of Health 2003). Despite a growing recognition of this dilemma, there is a governance problem at the heart of efforts to promote the public's health. Part of this lies in the nature of the public health system itself: large, diverse and without clear or fixed boundaries. But the issue is also a reflection of a preoccupation on the part of policy makers and managers, with acute health care services largely based in hospital. It is here, too, that the professional vested interests are at their most powerful and persuasive; the urgent forever driving out the important.

The root of the problem lies in the nature of the return on investment in health. Much of the investment in public health measures has a long-term impact and pay-off, whereas in the modern age of instant gratification and quick-fix solutions there is no incentive in investing for the long term. Politicians operating within a framework of short-term electoral cycles are driven to achieve quick, visible results. So treating more people in hospital becomes a *sine qua non* of success in health policy. The fact that as societies we are in many ways getting unhealthier seems to have escaped the attention it deserves. Instead, we blame individuals for the lifestyle choices they make and leave virtually untouched the powerful interests, such as those of the global food and drink companies, that certainly shape, if not determine, those choices (Hastings 2012). Yet, many of the 'choices' individuals make are constrained by policies emanating from central and local government, and by various industries as well as by various kinds of social inequality. The notion of individual choice determining health is too simplistic (Nuffield Council on Bioethics 2007).

To address this policy deficit, the governance issue is of paramount importance. As Wise and Nutbeam have argued: 'Our inability to reframe the role of health systems to include the promotion, protection and maintenance of the health of populations and to achieve a redistribution in countries' investment in their health sectors points to the need for significant rethinking of the approaches we have adopted to date' (2007: 23).

In any attempt to refocus health policy on health, there is a prerequisite to understand the key drivers and dynamics of modern health care systems. They are where the real power in the formation of health policy resides; a number of simple truths about health care systems demonstrate how extraordinarily difficult it is to shift the policy agenda away from them, as Wise and Nutbeam demonstrate. These simple truths can act as a brake on radical change and on shifting the paradigm from an ill-health to a health system. No matter how enlightened and visionary the policy frameworks may be, they will count for little if the mode of implementation is not addressed, and the need to disturb the prevailing power base is not accepted as an essential prerequisite.

What are these 'simple truths'? Five merit brief comment:

- *Health care systems want to grow.* Such systems are naturally expansionist and give rise to vested interests intent not merely on survival but on growth.
- *Higher health spending is believed to result in higher health status.* There are many fallacies and misconceptions in health policy but this must be among the most pernicious. Cross-national comparisons of expenditure and outcome reveal some puzzling patterns, with lower-spending countries as diverse as Japan and Cuba having better health status than higher-spending countries like the US. But, as the World Health Organisation (WHO) points out, it is the distribution of funds that may be a more important determinant of the success of a health system. There is no correct level of funding to allocate to health systems, although there may be a minimum per capita level – a baseline investment – below which health care is not going to be adequate (WHO 2000). The World Bank, in its global review of the relationship between spending on health services and population health (1993), concluded that although higher health spending should yield better health there is no evidence of such a link.
- *Universal access to health care does not lead to universally good health.* Such access has done little to change the way health status is distributed across population groups, with the wealthy continuing to remain healthier than those who are poor. Despite government attempts to close the health gap between social groups, inequalities have proved to be stubbornly persistent. Putting more resources into health care systems is therefore likely to widen the health gap unless a determined effort is made to improve the health of the poorest groups at a faster rate than the rest of the population. However, this is not a popular move politically so even when there exists such a policy its implementation remains weak.

- *Health care almost always wins out in the competition for resources.* Such an imbalance remains the case even when governments proclaim their commitment to improving health. This is because such promises are rarely backed by a significant shift of resources. Even when those resources are expected to be allocated to public health measures, it is not uncommon for these budgets to be raided to cover deficits in spending on acute health care, as happened in England in 2007. It is not difficult to understand why this should remain the case. Health improvement promises future not immediate gains, and it also challenges the status quo and the vested interests that profit from it. Whereas a shift from health care to improving health may strengthen social capital, the reverse may be true in the case of political capital. The public, fuelled by media scare stories of people's health being put at risk by a lack of resources or facilities, would not look kindly on politicians who failed to meet their perceived need for health care services.

- *Changing the distribution of health status through 'upstream' strategies is extraordinarily difficult.* Interventions intended to benefit the disadvantaged tend to benefit the already advantaged, thereby widening disparities and the health gap. Recent efforts in the UK to overcome this problem and meet targets by 2010 to increase life expectancy have resulted in the growing medicalisation of public health whereby hard to reach groups in local communities and neighbourhoods are targeted and prescribed statins and/or blood pressure lowering treatments to achieve quick wins in their health status and life expectancy. Such measures undoubtedly have their place but they ought not to be seen as a substitute for tackling the social determinants of health however complex and long-term the necessary commitment.

These 'simple truths' are reinforced by governments operating within increasingly short electoral cycles when in fact the health agenda demands a longer time horizon. So, caught between such pressures on the one hand and the vociferous demands of powerful vested interests on the other, policy makers find it extremely difficult to move upstream.

Almost every public institution and public policy sphere has health implications, which is why at the end of 2007 the Finnish government, during its presidency of the European Union, succeeded in getting the European Commission to adopt the concept of 'Health in All Policies' (HiAP). In its conclusions on HiAP, the Council of the EU calls:

> for broad societal action to tackle health determinants, in particular unhealthy diet, lack of physical activity, harmful use of alcohol, tobacco and psychosocial stress, since the individual capacity to control these determinants that account for major public health problems, is strongly associated with broader social determinants of health, for example the level of education and available economic resources. (Council of the EU 2006: Resolution 9, 3)

Moreover, health is largely determined by determinants outside the health care service. Therefore, HiAP is proposed as a strategy to help strengthen the link between health and other policies (Stahl et al 2006). It seeks to address the effect of health across all policies such as agriculture, education, the environment, fiscal policies, housing and transport through the use of tools such as health impact assessment. Through a HiAP approach, the wellbeing of countries becomes the responsibility not only of health structures, mechanisms and actions, but also of other sectors that may in fact have even greater influence on health and wellbeing. There is nothing especially novel about HiAP – it echoes WHO thinking enshrined in Health for All and earlier initiatives, notably the Ottawa Charter (1986) as well as the Alma Ata Declaration in 1978, which raised the profile of other sectors in health policy making. It is its revival in high policy-making circles that is significant at a time when health and wealth are seen to go together. Contemporary preoccupations with notions of happiness, noted earlier, and the health society are also directly relevant to HiAP. Not surprisingly, HiAP is a politically challenging strategy especially when health is largely constructed in other sectors beyond the health sector.

HiAP has its antecedents in an ecological view of health that emphasises that the contexts in which people live and the ways in which people relate to them are profoundly influenced by public policies. At a time when public policy is under threat from the neoliberal notion of the market state, HiAP is neither fashionable nor welcome in all quarters. If it is to survive, it will have to be fought for. The publication by WHO of a manual to provide a resource for training to increase understanding of HiAP by health and other professionals may assist in this endeavour (WHO 2015).

Two related policy paradoxes are evident in all our health systems and these cannot be ignored or overlooked. First, at the very time when public health is high on the policy agenda in many countries, its capacity and capability to deliver remain weak and fragile. Public health, or variants such as health improvement and wellbeing, is not regarded as central to health policy or institutionalised in the way health care services are. We already know a great deal about the social determinants of health. Indeed, the WHO Commission on Social Determinants of Health under the chairmanship of Michael Marmot makes the point that despite the vast majority of inequalities in health – between and within countries – being avoidable, action falls far short of what is required to tackle poor health among poor people and that the health gap is widening (Commission on Social Determinants of Health 2008). While technical solutions within the health sector are important, they are not sufficient. Dealing with the underlying causes and determinants of health may yield more significant and lasting gains. Importantly, the Commission argues that action on social determinants of health will empower individuals, communities and whole countries. But for this to happen, collective social action is a prerequisite. More generally, a social determinants approach 'seeks to redress the imbalance between curative and preventive action and individualised and population-based interventions' (Commission on Social Determinants of Health 2007: 16). It may not be widening so critically in some countries, but the general global trend is in that direction (Mackenbach 2005). We know, too, that modern illnesses such as obesity, lack of exercise, alcohol misuse, smoking, poor mental health, sexually transmitted infections, teenage pregnancy and so on are more evident among poor people than other social groups and tend to cluster in those groups over time (Buck and Frosini 2012).

This failure to arrest the growth of such modern pandemics constitutes the second policy paradox. It is well described by a long-standing health policy adviser in Finland, Kemmo Leppo, who says: 'One of the great paradoxes in the history of health policy is that, despite all the evidence and understanding that has accrued about determinants of health and the means available to tackle them, the national and international policy arenas are filled with something quite different' (quoted in Kickbusch 2007: 157). The policy dilemma facing us was neatly described by Wanless in his review of the state of public health published in 2004.

> Numerous policy statements and initiatives in the field of public health have not resulted in a rebalancing of policy away from health care (a 'national sickness service') to health (a 'national health service'). This will not happen until there is a realignment of incentives in the system to focus on reducing the burden of disease and tackling the key lifestyle and environmental risks. (Wanless 2004: 23)

After reviewing policy progress, or rather its absence, over some 30 years, Wanless concluded that the NHS remains a sickness rather than a health service, failing to shift the balance from health care to health. He suggested that the principal challenge lay in delivery and implementation and not further discussion or policy prescription. He also concluded that the public health workforce in its current state was not fit for purpose and that the poor state of the evidence base and lack of investment in research and development needed attention. Although, much to the amazement and delight of the public health community, Wanless did a great deal to reinstate public health as a major public policy issue, in practice, as noted earlier, little of substance has changed over the past decade or more. Indeed, the NHS chief executive referred to the lack of action in *The National Health Service Five Year Forward*

View strategy published by NHS England in 2014. Wanless took the view that has now become fashionable again a decade later that unless more was done to manage growing demand on the NHS it would become unaffordable and unsustainable. He was not alone in arriving at this conclusion. There is general agreement that no publicly funded health system is likely to be sustainable in the long term unless there is a significant shift in focus from ill-health to health. But although Wanless recognised this, he was far less certain that the government meant business. His initial gloomy assessment was confirmed in a subsequent review of progress undertaken for the King's Fund (Wanless et al 2007). Here, Wanless and colleagues concluded that too little progress was being made to tackle public health challenges such as obesity and that, unless there were a major shift in policy, the 'fully engaged scenario' he had proposed as offering significant improvements in health status that would eventually reduce expenditure on the NHS (see Box 3.1) would not be achieved by 2022.

Box 3.1: Fully engaged scenario: principal dimensions

- Levels of public engagement in relation to their health are high;
- life expectancy increases beyond current forecasts;
- health status improves dramatically;
- people are confident in the health systems and demand high-quality care;
- health service is responsive with high rates of technology uptake, especially in relation to disease prevention;
- use of resources is more efficient.

Source: Wanless (2002).

Without over-exaggerating, it can be said that the public health problems countries face – from obesity and alcohol misuse to rising mental illness, the commercialisation of childhood and environmental degradation – are outpacing the capacity of our institutions to change and meet the complex and deep-seated challenges posed. Our institutions and political systems appear to have become ossified and incapable of effecting the type and scale of change needed. They are, in management consultant speak, no longer 'fit for purpose' – if they ever were. Just as many countries have witnessed the rise of terrorism and asymmetrical warfare challenging conventional notions of war, our institutions have been overtaken by the pace of events and the global scale of the health challenges we face. 'More of the same' is no solution – that way leads to what Donald Schon (1973) terms 'dynamic conservatism', namely, a 'tendency to fight to remain the same'. If the primary determinants of disease are mainly economic and social, its remedies must also be economic and social. Yet, we invariably look to health care services to provide solutions. However, as the Commission on Social Determinants points out, in some instances health systems actively perpetuate injustice and social stratification, with health care resources being disproportionately consumed by the rich. The so-called 'inverse care law', first articulated by a Welsh GP, Julian Tudor Hart, is alive and well (Tudor Hart 1971). To this might be added the 'inverse prevention law': the greater the rhetoric around tackling the social determinants of health, the greater the policy emphasis on individual lifestyle change.

True health promotion is more than just a professional undertaking. It has the character of a social movement and can lead to radical change through engagement and collective action. The role of the individual as citizen rather than as consumer becomes central to the change process, as the next part of this chapter suggests. But there is a deep tension here that has been well expressed by McMichael and Beaglehole: 'Tension persists between the philosophy of neoliberalism, emphasising self-interest of market-based economies, and the philosophy of social justice that sees collective responsibility and benefit as the prime social goal. The practice of public health, with its underlying community and population perspective, sits more comfortably with the latter philosophy' (2003: 10). Yet, it is neoliberalism that remains in the ascendant, with all its negative implications for health (Schrecker and Bambra 2015).

Let us pause at this point to reflect on, and draw out, some key themes. Much of the difficulty facing health systems and the inability to change direction, except at the margin, lies in the government remaining wedded to a misconceived notion of what constitutes an appropriate response to the health challenges we face – what we have called the 'diseases of comfort'. Apart from being rooted in a medical model of health, many governments seek to control and impose from the top through elaborate systems of targets and performance assessment. This occurs even when the talk is of local autonomy, devolved responsibility and less central control. It is conceivable that the shift of public health back to local government in 2013 and away from the NHS might tackle some of these problems, but it is too soon to pass judgement and the pressures on local government from significant public spending cuts may make it impossible for it to deliver on the public health agenda.

Furthermore, much of the paraphernalia of modern management in public services is predicated on mistrust and on seeing professionals and the public as part of the problem rather than the solution. There is no real engagement between policy makers and the professionals on whom they rely for the implementation of their policies, or the public (or publics) whom the policy makers ostensibly 'serve'. Rather, attempts to involve the public are stage-managed, media-driven occasions devoid of any real meaning, substance or purpose. It seems that at least some governments, while often preaching the virtues of local action for its innovation and responsiveness, do not easily give up power but prefer instead to accrue more of it even when professing to do the opposite.

This is not to favour less government action; much of what has been described in this chapter actually demands more of it. Government does indeed have a key role to play in promoting health. A common complaint is that it has abnegated its important and legitimate stewardship function as it has become mesmerised by the notion of slim in place of big government with all its functions outsourced to the private sector or transferred to individuals to provide for themselves. The latter has occurred to a large extent in social care, where eligibility criteria have become ever more narrowly drawn with the consequence that growing numbers of people are required to fend for themselves. The idea of government offering strong leadership has given way to a more hands-off role conveyed by somewhat vacuous and meaningless terms such as 'enabling' and 'facilitating'. But what is actually needed is more government engagement rather than less, although not more of what exists now. The nature of the health challenges that countries face demands a quite different approach from that on offer in most places. Hence the need for a new paradigm as set out in the next section.

Shifting the paradigm

If we are serious about building a broad-based public health system in place of a narrow, rather reductionist and essentially biomedically centred health care system of the type on display in most countries, then a good starting point is the US Institute of Medicine's (2003) definition of such a system. The concept of a public health system 'describes a complex network of individuals and organisations that have the potential to play critical roles in creating the conditions for health. They can act for health individually, but when they work together toward a health goal, they act as a system – a public health system' (Institute of Medicine 2003: 28).

In short, making the whole greater than the sum of the parts is the goal to which policy makers should aspire. The problem is that many do indeed aspire to such a goal and are wholly sincere in doing so. Their rhetoric is also laudable. But all too often, that is all there is – nice words in abundance, but no real commitment to action and even less evidence of any in practice.

Central to the notion of a public health system is the reference to 'creating the conditions for health'. A problem with much public health thinking and practice, especially that rooted in a medical model of illness and disease, is that it focuses on deficits rather than assets. Public health has tended to focus on identifying the problems and needs of populations that require professional resources and high levels of dependence on health care and other services. Moreover, evidence-based public health is still dominated by a positivist biomedical approach to understanding 'what works'. It therefore results in policy development that in turn focuses on the failure of individuals and local communities to avoid disease rather than their potential to create and sustain health. Deficit models have their place, but the danger is that, coupled with the vested interests of those who subscribe to and actively promote such views, they dominate policy discourse to the neglect of asset models that have more to do with maintaining health (Morgan and Ziglio 2007; Hopkins and Rippon 2015).

The asset model draws on the concept of salutogenesis, which the sociologist Aaron Antonovsky (1987) adopted in his work on how some people manage stress and remain well. He sought to investigate the key factors that support the creation of health rather than the prevention of disease. Salutogenesis asks what causes some people to prosper and others to fail or become ill in similar circumstances. It looks for positive patterns of health rather than negative outcomes.

An assets approach to health directs attention to the resources that individuals and communities have at their disposal to protect against negative health outcomes and/or promote health status. These assets can be social, financial, physical, environmental or related to human resources (for example, education, employment skills, supportive social networks and natural resources). Assets can operate at the level of the individual, group, community, and/or population as protective (or promoting) factors to buffer against life's stresses. They can promote self-esteem and reduce dependence on professional services that may in fact do little to promote this kind of positive health outlook. Allied to the assets approach are the twin notions of capability and resilience. The notion of resilience – that is, the ability to cope in times of stress – is especially important and useful. There is evidence, too, to show that communities that are more cohesive and characterised by strong social bonds and ties are more likely to maintain and sustain health even in the face of disadvantage (Kawachi et al 1997).

The new governance, to which a paradigm shift paying more attention to health assets than deficits would give birth, comprises the following elements:

- a focus on healthy populations rather than healthy institutions (for example, hospitals);
- managers of health in place of health service managers;
- the pursuit of managerial epidemiology, namely, responsibility for the health of a defined population;
- a recognition of the importance of 'place-shaping' and the notion of 'liveability' for healthy communities.

Through such means, a system of governance would be created in which HiAP, as described earlier in this chapter, becomes a reality – an idea that is similar to Ilona Kickbusch's (2007) notion of the 'health society'. A consequence of the health society is a shift from entities that are clearly defined as health care organisations to an increased dependence on mechanisms that apply throughout society and which regulate behaviours and consumption patterns. It may be a cliché and a familiar piece of rhetoric, but, according to this definition, health is in fact everybody's business.

The needs of the collective are not the same as the sum of individual preferences. The principal role of stewardship and governance is the protection of the population's health. This is, and will probably always be, an essential role for government, but it must include intersectoral collaboration with the private sector and non-governmental organisations, and community involvement in decision making and action. Collective responsibility and action should not be abandoned in favour of a focus on individual choice and consumer models of health promotion and prevention in which it is all a matter of giving people information and advice to allow them to exercise informed choice. The growing marketisation of public policy in many countries threatens and weakens the legitimate stewardship role of government as the ties between individuals as citizens and the state become looser, more transactional and contingent, and replaced by individuals acting as consumers in a marketplace.

If we are truly to progress to a new balance between health and society, health policy needs to be realigned so that it is not regarded solely in terms of expenditure and consumption of health care services.

There is a need to be much more vigilant about separating out health care from health instead of using the terms interchangeably. Politicians need to talk more about health and less about health services and, importantly, mean it. How often at gatherings of political parties or in media interviews do politicians talk about health as distinct from health care and hospital beds? Improving health is always equated with building new hospitals! But these politicians may be acting perfectly rationally, since elections are not won or lost on matters to do with the public's health. On the other hand, the fate of politicians' electoral ambitions could be critically affected by health care matters and a failure to provide safe, accessible treatments.

Health cannot be produced by a single sector or group of professionals working apart from the communities they serve. It has to be co-produced, since it is by definition cross-sectoral and concerned with empowering communities either to take greater control of their health or to maintain those health assets that already exist within individuals and neighbourhoods. Despite governments in many countries acknowledging the need for joining up policy and management and working across organisational and professional boundaries both vertically and horizontally, success in these efforts has proved negligible. Instead of merely repeating the importance of cross-government or cross-sectoral working, there is a need to understand the barriers to change and to act accordingly. Introducing markets into health systems is unlikely to resolve the dilemma facing policy makers and practitioners. Only strong and effective governments, working with and through the public, can determine what sort of healthy society we want. For example: what degree of inequality is acceptable? How far can the health gap widen before governments come under pressure to reduce it? What price the pursuit of better health – at all costs or at some level to be agreed? What should the limits be to the consumption of health?

Such questions are central to what a holistic health policy should be concerned with. They cannot be satisfactorily addressed without agreement on the values that will ultimately drive the health society. This is why we need to adopt and implement an ecological model of public health that both recognises the importance of the whole system and the requirement to reconnect people with their health (Lang and Rayner 2012). Part of such a model includes a more vigorous critique of the notion of human 'progress', particularly one that is driven by economics and adheres to a particular conception of modernity and economic development. The new behavioural economics is beginning to offer an alternative narrative that embraces health and wellbeing. But the public health community needs to be more passionate about health issues associated with human progress and to adopt a vigorous health promotion stance. Its practitioners can no longer merely be dispassionate bystanders or analysts describing the problem. They need to become advocates for change. The NHS chief executive recognises this in *The National Health Service Five Year Forward View*, stating that the NHS will 'back hard-hitting national action on obesity, smoking, alcohol and other major health risks' and will 'advocate for stronger public health-related powers for local government and elected mayors' (NHS England 2014: 3).

Too often, people are helpless when faced with largely unhealthy choices. Public health should be leading the way, pointing out that diseases of comfort are an outcome of human 'progress' and civilisation, and ensuring that, through health-promoting education, built and social environments and legislation, comfort choices are healthy choices for all and not merely the few.

The notion of tipping points may be relevant here and could provide the trigger to usher in the new paradigm required (Gladwell 2000). Tipping points are social epidemics that spread through populations in much the same way viruses do. They can refer to socially undesirable as well as desirable behaviour, including binge drinking among teenagers, smoking among young women, or the falling crime rate in New York. Tipping points are a form of contagious behaviour and occur through small changes having big effects. As Gladwell puts it: 'the name given to that one dramatic moment in an epidemic when everything can change all at once is the Tipping Point' (2000: 9). A good example of such a tipping point is the ban on smoking in public places. Prior to Ireland taking such bold and decisive action in respect of healthy public health, which, in effect, constituted the tipping point, governments elsewhere were sensitive to the charge of the 'nanny state' and resisted taking action that could be so condemned. But what happened in Ireland had a ripple effect in respect of the UK, when it became clear not only that the policy seemed to work but that it enjoyed widespread public support. First to follow Ireland's lead in the UK was Scotland, which had been granted political devolution and its own parliament in 1999. The then First Minister for Scotland was so impressed by what he saw on a brief visit to Ireland that he returned determined to act on Scotland's appalling health record, to which high levels of smoking contributed. Losing little time, Scotland introduced the first UK smoking ban in March 2006 and its impact has been remarkable. The rest of the UK quickly came into line a year or so later, even England – where politicians were reluctant to act, nervous about being accused of acting like the 'nanny state'. But the important fact about this social movement or epidemic was that public opinion was in favour of the move and possibly ahead of politicians. This has been demonstrated by high rates of compliance with the new law and the acceptance, even among smokers, that public places are much more pleasant to visit as a result. Of course, smoking has not been eradicated and in some groups, notably young women, it is increasing, so a smoking ban is not an answer in itself. But the ban is a major step away from smoking being regarded as acceptable social behaviour. Had Ireland not acted, and had Scotland not followed soon after with its own legislation, it seems unlikely that similar action would have occurred elsewhere in the UK, and least of all in England. The ban, then, could be said to be an example of the kind of social epidemic to which Gladwell refers. There was certainly a contagious dimension to the way in which the smoking ban was embraced as the right thing to do at a particular moment in time and following Ireland's example.

Tipping-point thinking centres on improving receptivity to new ideas and to change. Often all that is required to encourage such thinking is simply to present information in new and different ways. Or it may be a case of identifying those individuals who hold social power and can help shape the course of social epidemics. In England, it took a celebrity chef, Jamie Oliver, to draw public attention to the poor nutritional quality of school meals. Largely as a result of a series of hard-hitting television programmes fronted by Oliver, which received considerable public attention, the government moved quickly to reform school meals and make them healthier. Almost overnight, a new policy was developed and implemented. Of course, not all parents approved of the changes, as graphically shown by newspaper pictures of mothers feeding hamburgers to their children through the railings of their local school. But they were a minority, albeit a vociferous one. The problem had been known for many years and public health practitioners had argued for the reform of school meals but nothing happened until Jamie Oliver's simple message captured parents' hearts and minds, and immense pressure was brought to bear on government not only to act but to be seen to be doing so – and quickly.

Creating the health society may therefore not be an entirely unattainable goal. Although the need for stepping up the pace of change is great, at least there is evidence from a few small examples that change is not impossible and can come from unexpected quarters. Tipping points may therefore be seen as a reaffirmation of the potential for change and the power of what Gladwell calls 'intelligent action'. There are important lessons here for the kind of public health system needed and the sort of skills required to engage with the public and to encourage them to seek change and to exert pressure on government where it has a role to play. After all, people acting individually can do little to influence powerful multinational food and drink companies. But acting together, and putting pressure on governments to act, can be a powerful force for change. That is why neoliberalism, with its emphasis on individualism and choice, has narrowed the focus of public health and is antithetical to most of what it stands for (Stuckler and Basu 2013; Schrecker and Bambra 2015).

Towards a health strategy for Europe

In response to the revival of interest in public health, the WHO Regional Office for Europe decided in 2010, on the appointment of a new regional director, to put public health back at the heart of WHO's activities. The rebalancing of its public health focus came to a head in September 2012 when WHO launched its new European health policy framework and strategy for the 21st century, *Health 2020* (WHO 2012a). It received the unanimous support of all 53 member states stretching from Iceland in the west to the Pacific coast of the Russian Federation in the east. *Health 2020* was accompanied by a *European Action Plan for the Strengthening of Public Health Capacities and Services* (WHO 2012b), intended to serve as the main implementation pillar for the strategy.

At the heart of *Health 2020* is a commitment to social justice and fairness and a conviction that current inequities in health across the social gradient are both intolerable and unsustainable. Moreover, they are seen to be the result of a 'toxic combination' of 'poor social policies and programmes, unfair economic arrangements, and bad politics' (Commission on Social Determinants of Health 2008: 26).

The goals of *Health 2020* are to achieve better health for the European region and its people, to increase health equity and accelerate progress on achieving the right to health, to make health an endeavour for all of society, to enhance regional and global awareness of and action for health and the determinants of health, and to develop solutions, tools, evidence, guidance and partnerships that support health ministries and other stakeholders in putting in place national policies, services and governance arrangements that realise their societies' health potential on an equal basis.

These are rather grand, if not grandiose, goals and much work is in progress to ensure that they can be made a reality, at least in some countries, if not all across Europe (Hunter 2012). The Regional Director, Zsuzsanna Jakab, believes that although *Health 2020* is 'complex and challenging, it is at the same time coherent and practical' (Jakab and Alderslade 2015). Yet it still faces a tough challenge. As we have seen from the UK's experience of improving health and reducing inequalities, the task has proved stubborn and difficult even where countries possess the means or resources to make convincing progress (Bambra et al 2011).

Several questions arise over *Health 2020* and what it is hoped will be achieved. Two stand out. First, why has WHO chosen this particular time to devise a new strategy when countries throughout Europe are grappling with huge economic problems and making deep cuts in public spending and services? What can it realistically hope to achieve in such a harsh, austere political and financial climate? Second, what will be different about the policy compared with earlier efforts that were criticised for being overly ambitious and rhetorical and for failing to be implemented?

On the first point, as was noted earlier, confronting the rise in non-communicable diseases entails difficult decisions both for governments and for individuals. These decisions are intensely political and raise questions about what governments regard as their legitimate role and purpose. The swing to the political right across Europe in recent years, coupled with economic hardship resulting from the global financial crisis of 2007-08, is being challenged, notably in Greece, where citizens elected a left-wing government in January 2015 opposed to further austerity policies. But for those governments on the political right, tackling widening health inequality and a growing health gap are not seen to be high priority or even a legitimate role for government. The view taken is that responsibility for health lies with individuals.

On the second point, earlier WHO health strategies, notably Health for All, have achieved little in practice while being widely cited. With *Health 2020*, WHO is acutely aware of the high expectations to achieve results. Yet, as a United Nations body, WHO can only work through consensus and unanimity and cannot force a government to take action. With *Health 2020*, WHO hopes to be able to persuade at least several member states to invest in prevention and shift the balance of health spending accordingly and to realise that tackling the growing health gap is vital to ensure vibrant and economically productive communities – a claim, as noted earlier, articulated in the UK by Derek Wanless (Wanless 2002, 2004).

WHO cannot act alone. It needs to operate in concert with other organisations active in the European Region. Working with the European Union (EU) will be important. The 27 EU countries comprising part of the WHO European Region have an integration and cooperation process in health based on the EU health strategy as well as policy frameworks and other mechanisms to implement these. Better integration between EU and WHO initiatives could contribute substantially to implementing *Health 2020*, although securing such joint working and aligning policies has proved problematic in the past.

Part of the difficulty here lies in the fact that the EU is essentially an economic idea that drives its various institutions with the possible exception of the European Parliament, although this is probably the weakest of the EU institutions. The problem may lie with the actual concepts of health and health policy and what they stand for. These are hotly contested notions. Are they about the allocation of scarce resource? Or about influencing the determinants of health in order to improve public health? Or about government policy for the health service? EU treaties are concerned with public health rather than with health care systems, although much of what happens in the EU beyond its public health interests directly affects health care systems, including the various rulings of the European Court of Justice in respect of people seeking treatment outside their own country of residence while expecting their own health service – which may have had a waiting list or may not have offered that particular treatment – to pay the costs.

The EU's central concern with economic matters means that issues associated with health and health systems tend to remain near the bottom of the agenda except when, as in the case of the internal market directive mentioned earlier, they are seen as commercially attractive and a source of major economic development with significant market potential (Hunter 2007). The notion that health systems contribute to social cohesion and social justice is of secondary importance whatever the rhetoric may state. Indeed, such concerns only receive serious attention if couched in terms that can demonstrate their contribution to economic development. In such a discourse, only one value seems to matter – a thriving European single market.

Such a reductionist and economically driven approach may account for why the development of a comprehensive health policy framework has not been achieved – mirroring, it should be said, the drivers evident within particular EU member states. It may also account for the lack of a focal point for health policy, with developments affecting health policy, such as the working time directive, emanating from other more powerful directorates within the European Commission. Having said this, Robert Madelin, director general for health and consumer protection at the European Commission, suggests the issues are more complex. In a lecture at the Royal College of Physicians in London he explained that 'behind the headlines that say Europe is about markets and competitiveness against social goods or public goods, the same European Council is adopting Healthy Life Years (the sustainable health and wellbeing of individual citizens) as a key performance indicator for its competitiveness agenda' (Madelin 2006: 493). He viewed this as a sign for optimism.

Ilona Kickbusch (2004) believes that the lack of serious attention paid to health policy in most countries affords an opportunity for the EU. The European Commission, through its work on public health, aims to protect and promote the health of European people. Health is a key priority for the Commission and, given its comparative neglect in most countries, Kickbusch believes an opportunity exists to develop it in a European context. Indeed, work on public health has been allowed to develop at a European level precisely because member states had rather neglected their public health systems. They saw no political risk in allowing the Commission to meddle in this undefined area of health to which they did not accord much importance. Their main concern was that the Commission should not interfere with countries' health care systems. Consequently, at an EU level, public health policies have been strengthened in recent years. Contributing to this development have been national public health scares around food safety (such as BSE, and foot and mouth disease) and an acknowledgement that health is a transnational issue. The EU is committed to promoting health and preventing disease through addressing health determinants across all policies and activities. Yet, despite the rhetoric of a social model lying at the heart of Europe, health policy and its content are arguably increasingly regarded as a form of commodification and there is little connection between health and health inequalities and macroeconomic and trade policy.

Despite its growing importance, public health policy remains weak within the EU's overall responsibilities. Indeed, other policies frequently contradict public health policies. A good example is the common agricultural policy (CAP) with its subsidies for food production, which may well contribute to poor health in terms of rising obesity in European countries. This is because the subsidies favour the production of beef and dairy products high in saturated fats (Birt 2007). We know, too, that shopping habits are influenced by the CAP in terms of which foods receive subsidies. Dairy and meat production are favoured over fruit and vegetables. More generally, in the enlarged Europe, there are major inequalities in evidence, including marked differences in mortality rates. Why should a Swede live up to 12 years longer than a Lithuanian? Smoking kills, yet some EU members disregard this fact. Why? And why is there a standardised approach in respect of the single internal market but not when it comes to public health, disease prevention, health protection and promotion? Why is health not seen as critical to the future of Europe's competitiveness in a global economy? Indeed, similar questions are being asked within EU member states, including in the UK, in the context of debates about happiness and wellbeing led by, among others, Richard Layard (2006) and the New Economics Foundation (2006).

One answer to these questions may lie in the way functions and policy areas are packaged and compartmentalised in the EU, each located in its own silo akin to the situation prevailing in most countries that make up the EU (although, interestingly, during its presidency of the EU, Finland made a point of integrating health into the work of other policy sectors and departments under an initiative known as Health in All Policies (HiAP) (Stahl et al 2006)). Health is generally seen as a narrowly defined organisational and policy sector – the health care system or public health system – and not an especially significant one at that. It is not regarded as a guiding value of European policy making that goes beyond seeing the EU as a common market to seeing it as a union that promotes the common good for Europeans.

If the latter were the norm, health and wellbeing would play a central rather than a peripheral role and would constitute a core value. Robert Madelin argues that progress is being made in this direction. Looking across the range of EU actions, it is possible to identify many areas that demonstrate that Europe is determining the parameters for some of the non-health drivers for health outcomes such as water, food safety and product safety. Moreover, the Treaty of Maastricht stipulated that a high level of human health protection shall be ensured in the definition and implementation of all European Community policies and activities.

Apart from being promoted through the EU and other bodies active in the European region, advocacy for *Health 2020* can be strengthened by working with civil society and by third sector organisations that deliver health services. There is a social responsibility role for the private business sector too in promoting health and wellbeing. The hope, therefore, is that *Health 2020* can be 'a powerful vehicle for collective action ... to enhance the health and wellbeing of future generations' (Jakab and Alderslade 2015: 171). But, in the end, it will be judged by how successful its implementation proves to be and on that the jury is firmly out.

Conclusion

As this chapter has tried to convey, the public health challenges to be addressed within individual countries, and within larger groupings like the EU, are invariably complex and far from being susceptible to easy or simple solutions. They are examples of what have been termed 'wicked issues' to which there is often no single or simple solution but rather multiple solutions involving individuals, communities and government at all levels working together in new alliances. Action is increasingly needed at the transnational level, since, as is evident in respect of the EU and its policy making, no single government can enact policies sufficient to tackle powerful global corporate interests. Tackling wicked issues also calls on the need for a particular range of skills and capabilities, since there is a need to work across organisational boundaries, engage a wide range of stakeholders, and influence citizens' behaviour. This is what WHO means by a 'whole of government' and 'whole of society' approach. But even where governments appear committed to take action to improve health and tackle the associated social determinants, progress has been faltering and generally unimpressive, and there is a propensity for 'lifestyle drift' to take over (Popay et al 2010). This has led some to conclude that doing anything about health inequalities, and narrowing the gap between rich and poor, is simply too hard or painful for any government to seriously contemplate (Mackenbach 2010). In short, the political will is lacking.

In such contexts, and when faced with tackling complex problems, public health demands a stronger mandate. It is not a mandate to pursue a biomedical disease model of health, but rather one that values positive health and works with individuals and communities to unleash their potential to create tipping points or social epidemics for change. Public health leaders need to be both de-skilled and re-skilled to work in this new paradigm. They also need to become more visible and vocal, and to be in a position to challenge the dogma surrounding concepts like 'progress', 'modernisation' and the inexorable penetration of markets in civic life when it comes to promoting health. All too often such notions end up destroying the very fabric of communities that is seen as so important in the creation and maintenance of health. This view is not negative or defeatist but realistic.

If healthy societies are to be secured, a new paradigm is needed. The ones that presently exist are not working and have patently failed to transform health care systems into health systems. Merely to advocate more market liberalism and choice in health and elsewhere, as contemporary political leaders are inclined to do, in the belief that somehow cherished values (such as traditional family values) will be preserved and reinforced is seriously to misunderstand the nature and dynamic of markets. As mentioned above, Sennett (1999) understands their corrosive effect on character and has written eloquently of modern capitalism's ability to 'radiate indifference'. In this paradigm, people are treated as disposable and 'diminish the sense of mattering as a person, of being necessary to others' (Sennett 1999: 146). Such features were not always present in capitalism but they are very much to the fore in its modern 'flexible' form. If the health society as described in this chapter is to take root, develop and flourish, capitalism and its accompanying neoliberal ideology need to be harnessed to, and play their full part in, a different ethic, one that values people's assets and builds on them.

A strategy of 'more of the same' is therefore not the answer and will no longer suffice. The outlines of what a new paradigm could look like have been sketched above. In particular, this ideal requires social movement thinking to achieve the desired action and change of direction, working with communities to enhance their sense of worth and self-esteem and, in so doing, to bring about real health improvement and wellbeing. Without a new paradigm to guide policy, what are increasingly sick societies are likely to get sicker.

FOUR

Models of health system reform

Introduction

This chapter describes and analyses the three phases, and contrasting models, of reform of the UK NHS that have occupied governments, principally key ministers and their advisers, from 1997 up to 2015. They have been articulated by one of the last Labour government's most influential health policy advisers, Simon Stevens, who labelled the phases as follows:

- benign producerism
- command and control
- new localism.

Stevens left his position as adviser to former prime minister, Tony Blair, to take up a new post as president of United Health in Europe, a major US health care provider, which over the years has competed for work in the UK, including providing general practitioner services in parts of the country. In April 2014, Stevens returned to the UK to take over as NHS chief executive. Although his phases of reform were developed during the Labour government's term of office, they remain relevant to the more recent changes introduced by the coalition government in 2013.

Britain is something of a market leader in health care reform, having been at it longer than most countries and with a determination and persistence not evident to quite such an extent anywhere else. One eminent commentator, Rudolf Klein, argued that although health care reform 'has been one of the worldwide epidemics of the 1990s ... Britain stands out from the rest' (Klein 1995: 299). Moreover, since 1999, and as is described later, post-devolution Britain has created growing interest as a laboratory for the study of differences emerging in the health systems taking shape in England, Wales, Scotland and Northern Ireland (Connolly et al 2010; Timmins 2013; Bevan et al 2014). As noted in Chapter Two, the reform path adopted in England is different in a number of important respects from that being followed in Wales and Scotland but especially in respect of its adoption under successive governments of market-style incentives, choice and competition in the use of the private sector, and in a separation of the commissioning of services from their provision. Developments in Northern Ireland have been slower to take off because the assembly was suspended for a time. The intra-UK differences in health policy are considered in more detail below in the final section to this chapter.

Before exploring the three reform models listed above, it is important to note that over the past 25 years or so, the governments of nearly every developed country have considered making major structural and institutional changes to their health systems. In his study of implementing change in health systems, Michael Harrison (2004) looked at the introduction of market reforms in the UK, Sweden and the Netherlands. All three countries, and some others, gave prominence to the development of market-like processes that would provide incentives for statutory insurers and providers to become more efficient and improve quality. Although quasi-market reforms had been introduced in the UK by the Conservative government in the late 1980s and 1990s, Labour entered office in 1997 committed to abandoning them. For a time, it gave the appearance of honouring its manifesto commitment. However, Labour was ultimately committed to a reform agenda similar to the Conservatives', having been persuaded by the prevailing orthodoxy evident both among its advisers (who, unlike their predecessors in previous governments, proved to be powerful shapers of policies and had the ear of their ministers – often in preference to the traditional senior civil servants), and among the international management consultancies on whom it had come increasingly to rely, that there was no other way. Indeed, so it was advised, the preceding Conservative government's cardinal error had been not to have the courage of its convictions and go far enough in the introduction of market-style changes. The Labour government did not make the same mistake, although it did not immediately seek to reinstate the virtues of competition and choice. Nor did it complete its work by 2010 when it left office to be replaced by a coalition government, which took over where Labour had left off. Between 1997 and 2015, when the coalition government came to an end, the reform agenda in England followed Stevens' three stages, which are described in the next section.

Health system reform in England

Benign producerism

First, there is the notion of 'benign producerism' whereby health systems are left largely in the hands of the medical profession. Since doctors effectively control the resources that get expended on health care interventions through their daily decisions concerning who does, and does not, get treated, it seems only reasonable to allow them the power to shape how health services are delivered. Consequently, in many health systems through the post-war years it was doctors who effectively were in charge. But this view was challenged and criticised for allowing doctors too much decision-making freedom and power. The term 'clinical autonomy' captured the essence of the problem. It was decided that doctors were insufficiently accountable for their freedom and that systemic problems arising from growing waiting lists and difficulties of access to care, especially on the part of some social groups, were the result of health care providers running services more for their benefit than those of their patients. Years earlier, Klein had described the British NHS as being in the grip of 'workers' syndicates' (1971). And Stevens posits that 'as well as being altruistic and principled', health care providers 'can also occasionally be inefficient, variable in quality, self-interested, and unresponsive to patients' preferences' (Stevens 2004: 38). Evidence for these failings could be found, *inter alia*, in the tragic events that occurred at Bristol Royal Infirmary where cardiac surgeons operating beyond their competence caused the avoidable deaths of many children (Bristol

Royal Infirmary Inquiry 2001) and later at Mid Staffordshire NHS Foundation Trust where patients suffered appalling care between 2005 and 2008 (Francis 2013).

Despite the many challenges to medical hegemony, it remains a live issue in contemporary health systems (Hunter 2006b). Even where it has been claimed that the power of the medical profession has been tamed or cowed, there remains a sense that such an interpretation may be too facile and that the medical profession's power lies dormant rather than curbed. Indeed, in the reassessment of the NHS reforms in England under Labour, a key element of the critique has been how the medical profession has been marginalised, if not altogether excluded, from the reform process, with the result that the changes cannot possibly work as intended. Instead of being regarded as the problem, the medical profession is now seen as part of the solution. With the appointment of an eminent cardiac surgeon, Ara Darzi, as a junior health minister (from 2007 to 2009), the Labour government appeared to have accepted this criticism and shifted its stance accordingly. Darzi was charged with leading a major year-long review of the next steps in the reform of the NHS. In an interim report, published in October 2007, Darzi observed that staff felt they 'had been ignored, that their values had not been fully recognised, and that they had not been given credit for improvements that had been made' (Department of Health 2007). He reported clinicians saying that 'they feel constrained and undervalued by managers', but balanced this by acknowledging that 'managers sometimes see clinicians as stubborn and slow to change' (Department of Health 2007: 49). A further brief progress report, in the form of a framework document setting out the principles for future change, was published in May 2008 (Department of Health 2008b). It set out five pledges for NHS organisations to observe when delivering change in their respective areas: change will always be to the benefit of patients; change will be clinically driven; all change will be locally led; change will involve patients, carers and the public; and existing services will not be withdrawn before new and better services are available to patients. Darzi claimed that future change was not about the way the NHS is funded or structured but that it must be about supporting local change from the centre 'rather than instructing it' and that health staff must be 'empowered to lead change' (Department of Health 2007: 49). There was also a commitment to making care fairer by reducing health inequalities, and making it more personal through embedding patient choice, already available in secondary care, and extending it to other areas such as primary care and long-term conditions.

Looking back it is not clear how much impact the Darzi review had following the change of government in 2010, although the rhetoric around putting 'clinicians in the driving seat' and setting 'hospitals and providers free to innovate' was central to the vision for the NHS articulated in the 2010 White Paper (Secretary of State for Health 2010b). Indeed, the White Paper had the words 'liberating the NHS' in its title. In that sense, there was considerable continuity between the dying years of the Labour government under Gordon Brown's premiership and the coalition government.

One of the many paradoxes of the Labour government was Brown's views about the NHS changes. Although he was one of the key architects of New Labour and the party's renewal and revival in the mid-1990s, he expressed strong reservations about the extent to which markets and medicine mix (see Chapter Six). However, it was not clear where he wished to draw the line in regard to how far market-style thinking and incentives could or should go in health care in England. There appeared to be an ambivalence and differences of view between him and Andy Burnham, his health secretary at the time, who was opposed to what he regarded as the growing marketisation of the NHS and wanted to enshrine the principle of the NHS as preferred provider in any contracting arrangements. Alternative providers would only be considered if the NHS could not deliver having been given every opportunity to do so. But this line was not upheld by others in the government who had no problem with a mixed market of service providers.

Command and control

If 'benign producerism' was criticised as a viable reform strategy, so was the second wave of health reform, which focused on top-down mechanisms and command and control models of centrally directed management systems. Such models had much in common with 'Fordist' thinking mentioned in Chapter Two. The belief that government can direct strategy, pull levers and get people on the front line of health care to do its bidding holds endless appeal for policy makers, especially those newly established in power and eager to make their mark. Health has always been at the centre of politics in many countries, and, even where policy makers might wish it were otherwise by decentralising and allowing more provider discretion and/or market influence, it has proved difficult if not impossible for those same policy makers to let go and withdraw from direct intervention in one form or another.

This second type of reform model underpinned many of the changes occurring in the UK and elsewhere in the 1970s, early 1980s and late 1990s, as well as through the 2000s. Despite the rhetoric of localism and letting go that underpinned the coalition government's reforms, these only came to fruition as a result of the government's sheer persistence and determination to impose changes in the face of widespread opposition from all quarters. The reform model was largely informed by the view that doctors had, in effect, to be brought to heel and that a countervailing force, in the shape of management, should be strengthened and enabled to do this. This was very much the ethos of the Labour years. The coalition government sought to distance itself from such a stance, insisting that its changes were about reducing layers of bureaucracy and freeing doctors and other health care professionals to get on with what they did best, unimpeded by pressures to meet numerous centrally determined targets and respond to a stream of central diktats. But paradoxically, in order to embed these notions, it was forced to adopt a command and control approach.

Although a few doctors have become managers in the British NHS, for the most part, health care, or what are increasingly being called health system (Timmins 2015), managers come from non-clinical backgrounds. In contrast to health services in the US, for example, NHS managers are for the most part graduates with degrees in arts and social sciences. When Roy Griffiths recommended the introduction of general management in the early 1980s, he assumed that many of the positions would be filled by clinicians (Griffiths 1983). Reflecting on his changes some years later, he was disappointed to discover that this had not happened (Griffiths 1991). Centrally planned and managed health systems came in for criticism, however, for being insensitive to the complexities of health systems and the need for them to remain flexible and adaptive to their particular changing needs and contexts as expressed by local communities. Micro-managing such a complex system from the centre was seen to be neither desirable nor appropriate even if it were feasible – which many doubted. Moreover, although ministers spoke the technocratic language of management, they remained politicians and there was a concern that the NHS was becoming more politicised, with managers more attentive to shifting political moods than to the needs of their organisations and services (Hunter 2000; Blackler 2006).

There was also concern that a uniform approach to change driven from a remote centre was inappropriate. For instance, the health needs of older people living on the south coast of England are quite different from those living in decaying inner-city housing estates. A 'one size fits all' approach was therefore not seen to be appropriate. A further problem with centrally planned and run health systems was the risk of continuous political interference and meddling, not only in the overall strategic direction of the health system, which was a legitimate function of elected politicians and ministers, but also in the means of achieving their objectives.

In recognition of these possible defects, there has been interest in England in putting the NHS under the control of an independent board along the lines of the BBC or Bank of England (Edwards 2007). The coalition government's changes introduced in 2013 (known as the Lansley reforms after their architect, Andrew Lansley, who was Secretary of State for Health at the time) sought to reduce the Secretary of State for Health's powers so that day-to-day managerial control was invested in a new organisation, initially called the NHS Commissioning Board and then NHS England. This body was to be a statutory autonomous organisation 'free from day-to-day political interference' (Secretary of State 2010b). In addition, Lansley sought 'to limit the ability of the Secretary of State to micromanage and intervene'. However, Lansley's successor as health secretary, Jeremy Hunt, has been a much more hands-on minister and keen to show that he is in control, which suggests that there has in practice been little change in the relationship between the political head of the NHS and its operational management. Having said that, much depends on the relationship between the health secretary and NHS chief executive. What marks the current NHS chief executive, Simon Stevens, out from his predecessors is that he has not had a traditional management career working his way up the NHS ladder. Indeed, for much of his career he has been steeped in the political machinery of government in the role of special adviser. This has given him a unique insight into the workings of government and his former insider status has equipped him with a set of particular skills denied most NHS managers.

What this brief review demonstrates is that it therefore seems inconceivable that removing the NHS from political control will ever be possible and that having a chief executive who is so intensely political, as Simon Stevens undoubtedly is, has actually, and however unintentionally, strengthened the politicisation of the NHS.

Given what has been said above, it is not difficult to explain the appeal of a command and control approach to policy makers and why the commitment to a hands-off approach and gradual change announced in the early days of the government in 1997 proved short-lived. Neither is it difficult to see why 13 years later, the coalition government failed in the end to convince anyone that it was committed to localism and a bottom-up change agenda. On entering office, New Labour made a commitment to no further 'big bang' reforms in the NHS, opting instead for a policy of incremental change and gradualism motivated by what worked, with evidence-based policy, rather than the whims and fancies of politicians and their advisers, driving any changes. At the time, it was a welcome and refreshing move on the part of a government that did seem intent on 'breaking the mould' and being willing to learn the lessons from history. For a short time, the government was true to its word, but a growing realisation, or acceptance, on its part that the NHS was a sicker organisation than had been acknowledged took hold and the government quickly changed tack. Leaving things to doctors and managers to sort out as best they could (as 'benign producerism' would have it) was no longer regarded as desirable. It was too high a political risk and a step change in performance was needed so that results could begin to be seen by the next election.

Therefore, around 2000, with the publication of Labour's 10-year plan for the NHS, *NHS Plan: A plan for investment, a plan for reform*, command and control came back into fashion with renewed vigour as the government struggled to 'save' the NHS and turn it around. With a forceful and dynamic health minister, Alan Milburn, and a prime minister who had also personally pledged to rescue the NHS, the government was committed to getting a grip on the service. With the announcement of the NHS Plan, the government made it abundantly clear that it was back in the driving seat with a vengeance. Not since the heady days of the Hospital Plan in 1962 were policy makers so convinced of the power and potential of central planning allied to a cadre of professional managers eager to do its bidding on the front line. These managers were a consequence of the introduction of general management into the NHS in the early 1980s following a review of the management problem conducted by the late Sir Roy Griffiths, then chairman of Sainsbury's (Griffiths 1983). Griffiths did not foresee his shock troops being used as instruments of central direction to quite such an extent (Griffiths 1991), but by this time, management had become politicised and politics had become managerialised to an unprecedented degree. No one spoke the technocratic language of management better than the prime minister (Tony Blair) or his then chancellor, later prime minister, (Gordon Brown). And the health minister at this time, Alan Milburn, was cast in the same reformist and managerial mould.

As essential underpinning for the NHS Plan, and to legitimate the significant injection of resources that the government planned for the

NHS, former banker Derek Wanless was commissioned to conduct a review looking ahead 20 years (to 2022) to identify what challenges the NHS could expect to confront and to assess whether a tax-funded system could still be affordable and fit for purpose (Wanless 2002). Wanless concluded that, despite the significant challenges that lay ahead, a publicly funded system of health care remained viable. In a far-reaching report, he pointed out that hand-in-hand with additional resources to make up for serious underinvestment, there needed to be a paradigm shift in the way health care was delivered and that in particular, as the last chapter pointed out, there needed to be far greater emphasis on prevention and public health initiatives.

Wanless presented three scenarios – solid progress, slow uptake and fully engaged – each reflecting different assumptions about the effectiveness of NHS performance and the health status of the population. Solid progress was a scenario of steady and significant improvement, with public health targets met, performance gaps closed and life expectancy continuing to grow fairly rapidly. The most ambitious, though most resource efficient, of the three scenarios was fully engaged; the least ambitious, though most expensive, was slow uptake. Not surprisingly, because of its potential for savings in the longer term, the government unreservedly supported the fully engaged scenario. Were it to succeed, Wanless estimated that by 2022, the government would be spending less on the NHS since people would be taking more responsibility for their own health and therefore the population as a whole would be healthier. As was pointed out in Chapter Two, although endorsing the fully engaged scenario, neither the Labour government nor its successor, the coalition government, succeeded in implementing it.

New localism

The third and final wave of reform bestowed upon the NHS proved to be the platform for the market reforms that many health systems have been attracted to – and which some have introduced – in recent years. Sometimes referred to as the 'new localism' or the 'localist challenge', it is derived from a belief that health services should be more responsive to users and patients and that since market mechanisms are geared to doing precisely this they should be actively encouraged in health services through notions of allowing new entrants to provide health care and stimulating a plural supply of services. There are many elements of 'post-Fordist' managerial thinking in 'new localism'.

The Labour government was stung by criticism that its command and control style of management was Stalinist and had resulted in a demoralised workforce. Despite the injection of significant new money annually between 2001 and 2008, representing an annual growth rate of around 7%, more than double the 'normal' growth rate, the feel-good factor that might have been expected to occur after such lavish spending did not materialise. Instead, an almost palpable sense of failure and alienation could be discerned. The government did not help its cause by constantly hammering home the message that there could be no increase in resources without reform, leading people to conclude that the NHS was riven with deep-seated problems that remained largely unresolved. There were also ill-conceived remarks about the deficiencies of the workforce and its innate conservatism and resistance to change. Above all, there seemed to be an implicit assumption that change and progress were somehow, and axiomatically, desirable ends in themselves without there ever being a clear or consistent narrative accompanying them detailing their purpose.

Regulated competition and markets were therefore seen as the optimal means of achieving both efficient and high-performing health systems. The introduction of foundation trust hospitals was another means of achieving more local control. Although remaining publicly owned assets, such hospitals would in future no longer be principally accountable upward to the Department of Health but outward to their local community through a board of governors elected by staff, recent patients and local communities. An independent regulator, Monitor, was appointed to oversee the viability and operation of foundation hospital trusts.

Despite the focus on localism, greater autonomy and devolved responsibility – perhaps most graphically illustrated by the NHS

CEO telling managers to 'stop Kremlin watching' and look out to their communities rather than up to the centre – the government, like all its predecessors and successors, found it extremely difficult to let go. Exercising a self-denying ordinance does not come naturally or easily to a government possessed of its own certainty and giving all appearances of being on a mission. Far from the new localism being local, it is in fact a hybrid of central direction wrapped up in local rhetoric; perhaps this is the most confusing message of all for staff and public to comprehend, especially in the context of the coalition government's emphasis on liberation and on locally led change with the centre's role restricted to facilitating that change. In practice, the opposite occurred with local NHS organisations coming under heavy pressure from ministers to do their bidding but in a context made more fragmented and confusing by the organisational changes.

What makes the present situation particularly interesting and somewhat puzzling is the introduction of choice and competition designed to make the NHS more responsive locally as well as allow new entrants to the marketplace to provide services. Indeed, this push for change that started with New Labour was given added impetus by the coalition government's changes. Building on the experience in social care, the government extended individual budgets to the NHS for people with long-term conditions. Such developments raise major issues about the future of the NHS itself as well as about central–local relationships. Chapter Six explores these developments in greater detail. Before reviewing what happened under the coalition government between 2010 and 2015, and the extent to which the NHS changes it introduced represented continuity with the Labour government reforms, we should pause and reflect on health reform during the New Labour years. It laid the foundations for all that has happened since.

Reviewing health system reform over the New Labour years

The various reform moves comprising the second and third phases described in the last section can be viewed as constituting a challenge to the medical profession's power and to the notion of benign producerism that had largely prevailed previously. More seriously, they were viewed by many health care professionals as an attack on the whole notion of craftsmanship and what it meant to be a professional providing health care and treating the whole person rather than mere body parts. Part of the challenge has taken the form of deliberately introducing tension into the provision of care to overcome a perceived and often-natural tendency towards inertia inherent in all human systems (Berwick 2002). What Stevens calls the search for 'constructive discomfort' characterised much of New Labour's NHS reform strategy. However, whatever the alleged successes emerging from such a strategy, there has been a heavy price to pay in the form of low staff morale and growing disenchantment with the reform process among all staff groups, most notably clinicians but also including many managers (Blackler 2006). None of these features has significantly changed since then. Indeed, as this chapter will show, they became more acute during the coalition government years and remain a cause for concern.

Having entered office committed to ending the internal market introduced by the conservative government in 1989, and having begun to do so in its formative years, by 2002 New Labour was quickly accused of reneging on its promises. It seemed to be a case of 'the internal market is dead. Long live the internal market!' But this left the government's natural supporters wondering, as many still are in terms of what the Labour Party represents following its resounding defeat in the 2015 general election, what the road map was, as it seemed to comprise a pro-business, market-style reform agenda that went far beyond anything that even the Conservative Party was prepared to contemplate at that time and for which New Labour had been elected, at least in part, to dismantle and replace. That a Labour government should even be contemplating, let alone actively pursuing, such a reform agenda was anathema to the majority of its natural supporters both inside and outside Parliament.

With the arrival of 'new localism', few in fact believed the government's commitment to a hands-off approach to health system reform, so there was little surprise when stories quickly circulated about the bullying and pressure that went on behind the scenes to ensure that local bodies conformed to the government's thinking and did its bidding. Such anecdotal evidence circulated for much of the life of the government and has certainly been apparent since around the turn of the century in 2000. A celebrated instance of such tactics being employed occurred in regard to the government's programme of independent sector treatment centres (ISTCs). Owned and run by private companies, all of which happened to be based overseas, 25 ISTCs had been established by 2005 with more planned alongside existing NHS facilities and contracted by the Department of Health to carry out routine day case or short-stay procedures, such as diagnostic tests, hip replacements and hernia removals. Controversially, in order to attract ISTCs, the government was obliged to set up an uneven playing field, or rigged market, between NHS providers and the private sector. Having established ISTCs, the government was determined that they should succeed.

Consequently, where PCTs expressed reluctance to contract with ISTCs for fear of putting at risk local NHS services or losing staff to the private sector, the government in effect forced them to do so. This was when the impact of ISTCs was little known and had not been subject to external assessment or evaluation. However, even when evidence began to appear suggesting that they might be a waste of public money and not the spur to service innovation and improvement that had been assumed, the government refused to concede that its policy was in any way flawed. Former health adviser Julian Le Grand, quoting Department of Health evidence, claimed that ISTCs were 'significantly more productive, with shorter lengths of stay and more innovative practices than their equivalents within the NHS' (Le Grand 2007: 110). But the all-party House of Commons Health Committee took a different view in its hard-hitting critique of ISTCs (House of Commons Health Committee 2006). The committee did not consider that ISTCs were necessarily more efficient or better value for money than equivalent NHS centres. Nor had ISTCs made a major contribution to increased capacity. Finally, their very existence could put at risk local NHS hospitals.

It is possible, though unlikely, that such conclusions, together with the change of prime minister, influenced the government's announcement in November 2007 that the number of new ISTCs was to be significantly reduced, and the contracts terminated in the case of some existing providers. The announcement was presented, at least in part, in terms of such centres having achieved what they were intended to, namely, serving as a cattle prod for the NHS and encouraging it to raise its game, and improve its performance and the quality of care, all of which had been achieved.

Although the government has always denied the charge of privatising the NHS by stealth, arguing that a big chunk of it in the shape of GPs operating as independent contractors had always been private in any case, there was growing unease at the way private health care was being promoted as the solution to the NHS's ills and, by implication, at the way traditional publicly provided services were, if not exactly reviled, deemed poor quality and/or resistant to change and therefore unfit for purpose. The mantra was that what worked was what mattered and that as long as the NHS remained publicly funded through central taxation, *how* services were provided and *by whom* mattered far less, if at all. It was a neat and superficially persuasive argument that persists to this day, with the most recent exponent of the argument being the chief health economist at the King's Fund (Appleby 2015), especially as it seemed to respond to public concerns about poor treatment and lack of respect for individuals. There was a sense, in keeping with new public management rhetoric as described in the Chapter Two, that somehow the private sector did things better, especially in terms of the front-of-house niceties that attended to the personalisation of care.

Few doubted the technical competence of the NHS or clinicians in general, notwithstanding some notorious cases of serious error, notably the Bristol Royal Infirmary (BRI) tragedy involving a number of fatalities in the paediatric cardiac surgical service, the deaths of hundreds of patients under the care of GP, Harold Shipman, and the more recent Mid Staffordshire NHS Foundation Trust scandal that occurred on Labour's watch and became the subject of two inquiries including a lengthy public inquiry (Francis 2013). But when it came to simple and rather basic things such as communicating with patients and having welcoming public areas in NHS facilities, the sense was that much improvement was called for. Although public support for health service staff, especially doctors and nurses, remained high (as is still the case), the government saw staff as a major block to reform. Moreover, incidents such as the BRI affair and the Shipman case confirmed the government in its view that no longer could the medical profession be relied upon to get, or keep, its house in order. The Kennedy inquiry into the deaths at the BRI made especially powerful reading (Bristol Royal Infirmary Inquiry 2001). It pointed to the 'insular "club" culture in which it was difficult for anyone to … press for change or to raise questions and concerns' (Bristol Royal Infirmary Inquiry 2001: 302). Furthermore, such a culture was not unique to BRI, but was widespread across the NHS. Similar concerns were to the fore in the Francis inquiry on the events at Mid Staffordshire. The inquiry into the Shipman affair was critical of the way complaints against doctors were handled and of the weaknesses in rooting out poorly performing doctors (Shipman Inquiry 2004).

Whether these high-profile cases of abuse and malfunctioning have led 'professional monopolists', to use Alford's term (1975), to see their power base significantly curbed in the face of the challenge from the 'corporate rationalisers' is unclear and the subject of some debate among researchers (Hafferty and McKinlay 1993; Harrison and Pollitt 1994). Recent developments would suggest that doctors are on the defensive and have had their power curbed. On the other hand, the medical profession did exceptionally well when contracts were negotiated and clinicians were required to give little in return. In particular, questions have been raised about why such a generous settlement was made to GPs and consultants without corresponding productivity gains being sought in return. In reviewing progress in implementing his 'fully engaged scenario', Wanless concluded that 'there is very little robust evidence so far to demonstrate significant benefits arising from the new pay deals' (Wanless et al 2007).

Returning to the events under New Labour and its reform strategy, the government's rediscovery of, and rapid return to, markets and competition was aided by a succession of special advisers who, without exception, were wedded to such notions. As well as Simon Stevens, two others stand out – Julian Le Grand, who succeeded Stevens, and Paul Corrigan, who was brought in as Alan Milburn's adviser and who, some years later, succeeded Le Grand as health adviser to Prime Minister Blair. Like all other advisers, these two academics, both unelected and unaccountable, owed their position to political patronage. They were examples of the growing power and influence of advisers that exceeded anything that had been evident in previous governments. Such individuals certainly had far more authority and visibility than traditional civil servants, and their direct impact on policy can be detected in policy statements, ministerial speeches and seminars given at think tank gatherings. They also enjoyed more clout than any so-called academic experts who remained committed to the core values, principles and structures of the NHS and who were dismissed as diehards from a bygone era and as insufficiently 'modern' to be taken seriously. Both Le Grand and Corrigan, albeit no longer occupying key positions as government advisers, continue to comment on policy developments and remain proselytisers for health reform along competitive market lines.

Enter the coalition government

Perhaps it was the novelty of having a Conservative–Liberal Democrat coalition government that provided a distraction from the policy changes that were unexpectedly and suddenly announced barely two months after the new government assumed office. Or perhaps it was because the prime minister, David Cameron, had promised no more top-down reorganisation of the NHS while in opposition and the public believed him. Whatever the reason, the default position was quickly adopted, with 'big bang' health care reform once more firmly on the agenda and a government dogmatically determined to see it through regardless of any opposition (Klein 1995; Hunter 2011). Even the coalition agreement did not prepare anyone for the tsunami of reform that was to overwhelm the NHS within months of the new government having entered office. The charge that the previous Labour government had subjected the NHS to major change paled into insignificance compared with what the coalition government was about to unleash on an unsuspecting public and an unprepared health system. The fact the government did not have a mandate from the electorate for the upheaval that ensued did not serve as a deterrent. The health secretary, Andrew Lansley, was a man with a mission, who had been preparing for this moment for six years during which he was the shadow health minister (Timmins 2012).

The ostensible purpose of the reforms was to liberate the NHS from its perceived shackles under the Labour government. Power was to be put back into the hands of patients and clinicians. This was to happen by ending the 'target culture', removing layers of management and numbers of managers, and giving frontline staff more freedom to determine their working practices. The changes were a response to concerns that the previous government had virtually strangled the NHS in bureaucracy through its top-down 'terror by target' regime and fixation on delivery, accompanied by endless regulatory mechanisms and requirements together with an insidious bullying culture. Indeed, the decade from 1997 to 2007 witnessed the emergence of 'the audit society', with its avalanche of targets, performance indicators, league tables and reviews of various kinds (Power 1997).

An irony of the 'big bang' reform approach is that changes designed to liberate the providers and users of health care were imposed on them through the very top-down, command and control mechanisms that the government was at pains to dismantle and consign to the overflowing dustbin of failed reforms. Certainly, the reaction to the changes was unfavourable. And while the government tried to deny that its changes were about structure and instead sought to drive cultural change, in reality the structural changes proposed were considerable. Indeed, the NHS is still struggling to come to terms with many of them. The theme of cultural change was not new, but successive governments seemed unable to achieve it without meddling with structures. Moreover, dismantling and assembling structures has a seductive appeal and gives the semblance of change because, in contrast to cultural change, it is visible, tangible and can be achieved reasonably quickly according to fixed dates. Bringing about cultural change is a much longer-term and somewhat unpredictable enterprise that runs counter to short-term political and managerial time-frames (Braithwaite et al, 2008).

Three particular features of the reform proposals unveiled by the coalition government stand out. First, at no time during the general election did either of the two parties that subsequently formed the coalition give much of a clue about its intentions. Some of the Conservative Party's thinking was set out in general terms in policy documents and speeches, but attracted little attention during the election campaign. And as noted already, the Conservatives in opposition had rejected further major top-down structural change on the grounds that it was costly and did not work, and that the NHS had already been subjected to repeated structural changes.

Second, although the changes amounted to a big bang in terms of their impact on, and consequences for, the NHS's structure, they also represented remarkable continuity with the direction of reform set in train by the Labour governments under Blair and, to a lesser extent, Brown. What the coalition government did was apply greater resolve and determination to transform the NHS along the lines Labour had already mapped out in respect of the adoption of market principles of choice and competition. Had Blair been able to do so and had not encountered opposition to the proposed changes from his own backbenches, he would have gone further than he did.

Third, and perhaps most puzzling of all, is that it was never clear what the problem facing the NHS was to justify such an upheaval. At the time, all the indications were that the NHS was performing well and got high satisfaction ratings from the public. As Timmins (2012: 18) observed: 'the coalition government's upending of the NHS in 2010 came not amid an NHS financial or performance crisis but after the longest period of sustained spending increases in its history'. As was pointed out in Chapter Two, the Commonwealth Fund had given the UK's NHS top ranking overall out of 11 health care systems (Davis et al 2014). Why the government chose to expend so much of its political capital on a massive piece of legislation – the Health and Social Care

Bill – which was heavily opposed by all the health care professions and Royal Colleges and by those members of the public who had an inkling of what was going on remains a puzzle. Media coverage of the changes was generally rather poor and failed to get to grips with the key issues becoming lost in the welter of technical detail. Many MPs also found it difficult to get to grips with the purpose and impact of the changes, and this may have been the very reason why the changes could not be halted. Or perhaps it was because the new government could not afford to lose face and appear incompetent by confessing to a monumental misjudgement, preferring instead to plough on regardless and implement its ill-conceived changes. Or there may have been a more political and ideologically motivated reason, namely, that the architects of the reforms were fierce supporters of the neoliberal project to shrink the state. The coalition government could never admit to this in public, but nevertheless it may have been a key factor in its calculations to press ahead with the changes. We return to this explanation in Chapter Seven.

Twenty years of continuous change: a triumph of hope over experience

Much has been written about the various health reforms of the past 20 years or so. It is not the purpose here to rehearse the various arguments in detail, but to identify a few critical themes that appear to be common to various reform efforts and to query why governments of all persuasions seem attracted to particular types of change that often have no, or at best weak, evidence to justify them. What the various changes have in common is a focus on market-style competition and choice, the assumption being that while the funding of health services should remain in public hands, the provision of care may be public or private (including for-profit and not-for-profit arrangements). What matters is what works, rather than who provides what. The motives underpinning the various political parties' attraction to similar types of change, however, possibly do differ. For Labour, it was a matter of efficiency, effective management and delivery, while for the Conservatives and a wing of the Liberal Democrats (known as the 'Orange Bookers' after the Orange Book, which was published in 2004 and emphasised the role of choice and competition in public services), it was a matter of enacting a neoliberal commitment to small government and reducing public spending in the belief that an inflated public sector crowded out the private sector. Despite the motives conceivably being different, the direction of reform adopted by all the political parties was consistent, thereby allowing Simon Stevens to say of the coalition government's proposals that what made them so radical 'is not that they tear up that earlier plan. It is that they move decisively towards fulfilling it' (Stevens 2010).

While a return to any so-called golden age of first-phase reform in the shape of 'benign producerism' remains remote, at the same time no longer can reformers simply ignore the producers of health care or cavalierly disregard their views and concerns. Since the late 1990s, governments have by and large done exactly that and it has proved disastrous in terms of relationships between those providing health care and their political masters (in the main) and occasional mistress. Though doctors may no longer occupy the dominant position among Alford's structural interests, they certainly remain powerful and influential and a force still to be reckoned with, however much politicians may wish it were otherwise. Unlike those same politicians, doctors also continue to receive widespread public support. It would be premature to dismiss doctors and other professional groups as having completely lost their power and influence. Indeed, a long-standing observer and analyst of professions cautioned against making premature judgements of this nature. 'In the case of prophesying, or projecting, trends into the future, due caution requires being aware of the danger of mistaking short-term, ephemeral trends for long-term trends and cyclical change for linear, progressive change' (Freidson 1993: 57). Taking a long view therefore seems prudent.

While much of the discussion presented here of health policy over the past two decades or so is highly critical of successive governments' attempts at, and chosen instruments of, reform, it is only fair to balance this with an account of what has gone well and of those initiatives that have been long overdue. In particular, the acknowledgment in the late 1990s that the NHS was seriously underfunded was an important step in refurbishing the NHS and arresting the decline in its physical appearance that had become evident during the years of the Conservative government. Under the coalition government, that commitment to maintain and possibly increase funding in the face of an ageing population and its growing demands on the health system, and in the midst of a political fixation on austerity, is lacking, with the consequence that we may be witnessing a repeat of what happened in the late 1990s. This time, however, the neoliberal ideology at the heart of the current Conservative government's agenda has been given a new lease of life, with further cuts to public spending and welfare in hand.

Back in the late 1990s, there was also a commitment by the then Labour government to tackling child poverty. While the aim of abolishing child poverty altogether proved too ambitious, progress was made between the late 1990s and 2010, with the number of children in poverty falling from 3.4 million in 1998–99 to 2.3 million in 2010–11. Those gains have now gone into reverse, with the number of children in poverty rising since 2011. This reversal coincided with the coalition government's austerity measures involving deep cuts in public spending and welfare benefits. As noted in the last chapter, the gap between rich and poor is growing.

The tragedy for many critics of the Labour government's overall record of NHS reform is that these and other important developments – including the determination to improve the quality of care through levers such as clinical governance, evidence-based guidelines, national service frameworks for a range of conditions costed and based on robust evidence, and the arrival of the National Institute for Clinical Excellence (NICE) in 1999 – became largely overshadowed by a growing preoccupation with constant structural change combined with a fixation on markets and competition as the principal means by which its objectives could be achieved. The government squandered the opportunity it had to devise a reform strategy that genuinely learned from past mistakes and successes. As a result, as the official historian of the NHS, Charles Webster, put it, it 'seemed to fall into the same errors as its predecessors' (Webster 2002: 256). In particular, and repeating the mistake of the preceding Conservative government, New Labour vested 'unwarranted confidence in structural overhaul ...' and modernisation policies based on the new public management thinking described earlier.

As things turned out, these lessons were also ignored by the incoming coalition government in 2010, whose changes were entirely structural despite claims to the contrary. Moreover, in its attempt to strip out layers of bureaucracy (notably primary care trusts and strategic health authorities), the government actually rendered the structure more fragmented such that integrated care is now all but impossible. Part of the problem lay in the various changes and concessions that were made while the Bill was passing through Parliament before being enacted in 2012. But the government's own flawed analysis of what it saw as the solution to the perceived monolithic, overcentralised ethos of the NHS was responsible in large measure too. Lansley, in a previous ministerial posting, had been involved in utility privatisations. He believed the NHS could be run along similar lines if the conditions for a market akin to the utilities could be put in place. He believed that maximising competition in the NHS would improve services for patients, although there was no strong or convincing evidence to support such a view. But it was his conviction that new and independent providers should be encouraged to supply NHS care that lay at the heart of his proposals.

In every wave of NHS reform, a constant factor has been a tendency to ignore inconvenient evidence about the flaws in pursuing structural change and a wilful determination to put political ideology first. Of course, that is the right of elected governments, although whether any government elected on a minority of the popular vote has a clear mandate to pursue sectional interests to such a degree as the coalition government did, and its successor Conservative government has indicated it will do, is arguable. Why governments remain wedded to market-style notions of competition and choice and to the outsourcing of public services when the available evidence is less than convincing is something of a puzzle. Apart from anything else, it contributes to a perceived policy incoherence and lack of alignment.

Policy incoherence

If by 2002 there was a reasonably clear direction evident in the Labour government's health system reforms in favour of markets and competition, the precise means of achieving these reforms gave cause for concern and seemed to lack strategic coherence. In particular, the chief components of the new policy did not all mesh together in a coherent manner but seemed to push and pull against each other. The components were:

* private finance initiative
* payment by results
* practice-based commissioning
* plurality of providers
* patient choice.

Internal contradictions among these so-called 'jigsaw' policies, or 'five Ps', were rife (Hunter and Marks 2005; Paton 2006). For example, if the policy was to treat people in the community and out of hospital wherever possible, having a payments system whereby the survival of hospitals was determined by the volume of patients they treated seemed to introduce a perverse incentive. Instead of treating fewer patients, it was in hospitals' interest to attract as many patients into their beds as possible and given them as much treatment as possible unless, that is, those hospitals were to diversify their portfolio of activities and offer primary care and/or after-care services in a vertically integrated model of care. Although no hospital has so far seriously gone down this road, it is not inconceivable that some might, especially if their very survival is at stake. As we show later, new models of care are being actively encouraged as a result of the NHS Five Year Forward View (NHS England 2014).

To take another example of the confusion and incoherence at the heart of government policy at this time, if PCTs were being strengthened to become more effective commissioners for the health of their populations, how did this square with the emphasis on patient choice? Whose choice would prevail at the end of the day? Was it to be the PCT's or the patient's? Finally, to take a third example, while encouraging a plurality of providers may be attractive in boosting innovation and new models of care, what about the emphasis on collaborative, whole systems working and on joined-up policy and management in order to achieve seamless patient care? Encouraging diversity among providers risked an increase in fragmentation and a lack of integrated care. Indeed, such an outcome seemed especially likely in a mixed public–private market where issues of commercial secrecy might arise to prevent the free flow and exchange of information among all stakeholders.

Moreover, it was also unclear how commissioning by PCTs squared with the encouragement being given to GPs to become commissioners under practice-based commissioning (PbC) (Marks and Hunter 2005). While PCTs remained legally responsible for managing finances, for negotiating and managing all provider contracts, and for the overall commissioning strategy, PbC was intended to give general practitioners direct financial control of the way that health care is organised and provided. PbC could be undertaken by a single GP but was usually undertaken by a consortium or cluster of practices or by localities. Under PbC, practices could hold an indicative budget on behalf of their patients within which they would be expected to operate. Practices could commission services from, and manage referrals to, secondary and tertiary providers.

PbC was regarded as one of the central planks of the NHS reforms. Its purpose was to encourage GPs to have a direct stake in commissioning services and not withdraw from the process altogether, which larger and merged PCTs encouraged them to do since few wanted to be part of what they perceived to be bureaucratic health authorities. PbC was first mooted in 1998 and given a boost in 2005 as part of the most recent round of NHS changes. The Department of Health envisaged that by 2008 most practices would be engaged in PbC. This seemed rather optimistic as there was little marked enthusiasm on the part of GPs to become commissioners, especially as they were to be given only indicative, in place of hard, budgets while PCTs continued to hold the purse strings and oversee PbC. GPs could foresee a lot of additional bureaucracy for little apparent gain (Audit Commission 2006 and 2007). Perhaps their reluctance to become commissioners can be understood when set against a context of having been subjected to nearly 20 years of constant change in respect of primary care commissioning (see Box 4.1).

The coalition government in 2010, as we have seen, introduced a further raft of changes, thereby continuing and reinforcing the theme of policy incoherence while simultaneously seeking to simplify the NHS structure and give it a sharper focus centred on empowering frontline commissioners in the shape of GPs and Clinical Commissioning Groups (CCGs), which replaced PCTs. The intention was that CCGs would overcome the weaknesses evident in PbC and give GPs real budgets to improve health care for their populations. But the move was largely a structural one and did little to address the concerns among GPs, already noted from the Labour years, that most did not want to be commissioners of care or hold budgets. But what has also become more evident is that the fragmented, bureaucratic structure imposed by the coalition government has made it much more difficult for the NHS to deliver integrated care between primary and secondary care services and between health and social care.

Box 4.1: Primary care commissioning initiatives

1990–96	GP fundholding; total purchasing pilots: GP-led commissioning with health authority purchasing
1996–97	Locality commissioning pilots
1998	Primary care groups
2000	Primary care trusts
2004	First PbC guidance issued

Source: Audit Commission (2007).

Of course, the charge of policy incoherence and confusion in respect of the various governments' health system reforms has been vigorously denied by government supporters. For instance, former health adviser

Julian Le Grand, acknowledging the charge of incoherence and of introducing 'a contradictory mish-mash of ill thought out policy gimmicks with little basis in theory or practice', goes on to mount a brave if unconvincing defence of the Labour government reforms by arguing that they did indeed stem from 'a well-grounded understanding of the problems involved in delivering public services and, in particular, the difficulties in delivering them through forms or models of service delivery that did not involve elements of choice and competition – including trust, command-and-control and voice' (2007: 3). As a defence of what the government sought to achieve through choice and competition, this seems rather weak and to duck the central issue. It does little more than reiterate the view adopted by advocates of new public management that public services are no different from private businesses and should be subject to the same, or similar, disciplines in the shape of performance measures and incentive mechanisms. It has nothing to say about the special role of professionals or why public services may legitimately be subject, and managed according, to a different ethic and set of success criteria.

In any event, the Cabinet Office remained unconvinced by the last Labour government's NHS reform strategy. The contradictions and concerns noted above underlie the highly critical capability review of the Department of Health that the Cabinet Office produced in mid-2007. The review was especially critical of the lack of leadership at the top of the department and of the failure to convince either its staff or those in the field of the purpose of the changes and how they related to each other. It concluded that the department had not set out a 'clear articulation of the way forward for the whole of the NHS, health and well-being agenda' (Cabinet Office 2007: 18). It was not surprising, therefore, that staff and stakeholders were similarly unclear about the vision and felt little sense of ownership of it. Compounding the problem was a lack of any sense of the department as a corporate entity and a perception that it operated 'as a collection of silos focused on individual activities'. Its staff possessed 'a strong public service ethos, but corporate behaviours are weak' (Cabinet Office 2007: 18).

The department's change management strategies left much to be desired as well. It managed change poorly, 'placing too great a focus on structural change and headcount reductions' (Cabinet Office 2007: 19). Finally, the report was critical of the absence of policy coherence and the lack of integration among policies. Rather, 'policies tend to be developed in organisational silos and cross-boundary integration issues are not routinely thought through. Sometimes insufficient attention is paid to the impact these issues will have on delivery agents' (Cabinet Office 2007: 21). The result has been poor implementation, with stakeholders in the NHS and beyond wondering if, in keeping with Sennett's point mentioned earlier, policy makers were simply behaving like compulsive consumers of policy – a view given some credence in the assertion that the department 'generates too many initiatives without properly considering the interactions or offering any clarity on prioritisation' (Cabinet Office 2007: 19).

None of this came as a surprise to those observers who had made similar criticisms at the time the reforms were introduced. But in a seemingly high-handed way, which is the subtext of the Cabinet Office's capability review, the department chose to ignore such criticisms as the uninformed ravings of reform detractors who simply wanted the NHS to remain unmodernised and to be returned to a mythical golden age. The review urged the department to consider the need for more consistent engagement with frontline staff, 'enabling them to make an effective contribution to the development of policy and build common ownership of outcomes' (Cabinet Office 2007: 22).

While the capability review states what many detractors from the government's reform agenda in the NHS and wider public health arena appear to regard as 'the bleeding obvious', major questions arise over whether the department can, or in fact wants to, change direction and over the pursuit of its reform agenda. Subsequent changes of government have not heralded a substantive change of direction. This is because the changes that occurred in the machinery of government under New Labour go deeper and can be traced back to its arrival in government in 1997. When New Labour came to power in the UK in 1997 following 17 years in opposition, it did not consider that the civil service could be relied upon to provide neutral advice when it came to the development and implementation of new policy. Advisers, rather than civil servants, came to be regarded as 'their natural partners in government' (Cabinet Office 2007: 25). The growing reliance on consultants, which has continued unabated to this day, reflects this suspicion and distrust of traditional civil servants.

The impact of such a development is well analysed in Greer and Jarman's (2007) study of the changing Department of Health. In it they show how the department is NHS-dominated, with a strong managerial ethos, much of it supplied by management consultants on short-term contracts or on secondment from their firms, and with little civil representation at the top. More than any other department, they assert, 'it is the Whitehall that government want. It is one of the purest products of the delivery-oriented, businesslike "new public management" that has been orthodoxy in the UK since the 1980s. Relative to the other departments, it is focused on "delivery" rather than policy analysis …' (Greer and Jarman 2007: 7). The makeover of the Department of Health is the outcome of a long process in which, despite its title, the management of the NHS has come to be more valued than the broader remit of health. As the researchers state, the Department of Health

> is now as turbulent as the NHS because, like the NHS, it is a victim of media-driven policymaking and the plasticity of much English public administration. And that almost certainly means that the organisation and staffing of the DH itself has contributed to the confusion and contradiction that marks much health policy today. (Greer and Jarman 2007: 31)

Compounding the problem is the fact that the department is 'incessantly reorganising, and quite possibly is too willing to take on the implementation of political decisions that cannot be implemented' (Greer and Jarman 2007: 7).

In a subsequent critique of the coalition government's changes, the same authors find 'an unstable world, where the tensions between policy, politics and management of the NHS in England are likely to mean further reorganisation in the future, but with a "thin" central Department of Health less able to steer the system than before' (Greer et al 2014: 3). In particular, the separation of policy and management between the Department of Health and the NHS has never succeeded despite the efforts of successive secretaries of state going back to the early 1990s. With Simon Stevens' appointment as NHS chief executive, a blurring of policy and management rather than a clear separation between the two seems far more likely given Stevens' well-honed political antennae. At the same time, the current Secretary of State for Health, Jeremy Hunt, has shown no signs of wishing to relinquish his political leadership role of the NHS. Nor is he likely to be able to even if he so wished. As Greer and colleagues note, 'it is governments and politicians, not civil servants or agency chiefs, who are held accountable for their health policies' (2014: 20).

As we have noted, much of the policy confusion and contradiction identified both by Greer and Jarman and by the Cabinet Office capability review have their origins in the over-consumption of policy – an affliction that persists to this day. Rather than evidence-informed policy, there have been numerous reforms driven by ideology and conviction politics derived from a neoliberal agenda and set of accompanying theories. These have combined with a heavy, and growing, reliance on external consultants, many of them brought into government direct from multinational conglomerates such as McKinsey's and PricewaterhouseCoopers, who are among the principal beneficiaries of what Craig has called 'the golden years of management fashions, fads and quick fixes' (2006: 235). The most lucrative period in consulting was, according to Craig, the 1990s, when the government embarked upon a major public sector reform and modernisation programme that included, but was by no means confined to, the NHS. This was the period of over-consumption of policy, as described above, and an era marked by following the latest management fashion.

A major role of civil servants was to put a brake on policy ideas based on political whims and desires and to challenge ministers. In the new-style Department of Health, heavily staffed by advisers appointed by politicians, and managers on short-term contracts whose job is to do ministers' bidding faithfully, there is no challenge to the reforms being foisted on the NHS and these is a disregard for any notion of consensus building among stakeholders. The job of the new incumbents of the department is to focus solely on delivering political objectives rather than to undertake policy or risk analysis.

The fact that it the department is weak in analytic skills and policy research capacity is of little consequence and is in keeping with the prevailing politicisation of all policy. In such a climate it is hard to see how the hard-hitting critique produced by the Cabinet Office can have any impact or be addressed in the absence of any attempt to reverse the direction of travel that has been pursued so vigorously over the past two decades or so by successive governments. In the midst of the confusion and muddle that is almost endemic in contemporary health policy in England, it is often difficult to separate reality from rhetoric. For example, in their denial that they were (or are) privatising the NHS, successive governments have sought to reassure critics that they favour a 'third way' between traditional NHS providers on the one hand and for-profit providers on the other. Certainly the Labour government in the 2000s actively sought to encourage the development of social enterprises as alternative providers of health and social care services, even going so far as to establish a social enterprises support unit within the Department of Health. It claimed that such organisational forms were examples of true socialism, with their origins lying in the cooperatives, mutuals and related structures dating back to the 1920s and the era of 'guild socialism'. Similar attempts to expand the third sector were made by the coalition government in its efforts to stimulate a market in health care. It was sensitive to the charge that it was only interested in opening up opportunities to provide health care services to those who had donated handsomely to the Conservative Party or to businesses that offered lucrative directorships to retiring health ministers. But while there has always existed a niche for social enterprises, especially in respect of long-term conditions and chronic care, to expect them almost overnight to take over large tracts of NHS provision seemed naive in the extreme.

But, as in so much of New Labour thinking, there was a corruption of the original meaning of guild socialism. As a study of social enterprises in the NHS suggested, use of the term in the context of public service reform 'is becoming disconnected from its roots in the cooperative movement, community-focused businesses and local regeneration activities' (Marks and Hunter 2007: 50). At the same time, from on original emphasis on social regeneration and sustainability, the discourse has moved to embrace entrepreneurship, leadership and the application of business approaches to socially useful endeavour, and from providing care in disadvantaged neighbourhoods to providing choice through diversity.

Much is expected of social enterprises as a cure-all for many of the perceived ills of public services such as the NHS. Innovation, flexibility, nimbleness of response, and services close and more attuned to what people want all figure prominently. Yet, in a further example of policy incoherence, such expectations give rise to numerous concerns and contradictions. For instance, collaboration and 'whole system' responses to complex health needs might be rendered more difficult in an increasingly commercial and contractual environment. Decision making could also be slowed down by the introduction of bureaucratic arrangements for accountability. The notion of services being responsive to the local community could get lost in the search for viability in a competitive market or, more likely, through services being provided by multinational conglomerates without a local presence and with no desire to acquire one (Marks and Hunter 2007).

This last point is a real worry, since the fear is that many fledgling social enterprises would remain too fragile and unable to survive and would therefore be vulnerable to takeover by for-profit providers and over time become indistinguishable from such structures. Looking outside the UK, Borzaga and Defourny (2001) in their study of social enterprises across Europe point to a number of potential weaknesses. Marks and Hunter report these as follows:

one is the tendency for social enterprises to evolve into new organisational forms which serve to limit the original innovative characteristics which constitute their appeal. Another is the high governance costs which derive from their character as 'organisations without well defined owners' and their limited size, given links with local communities....They also point to a number of barriers, including that contracting out practices tend to favour large companies. (Marks and Hunter 2007: 50–1)

As a final comment, it is also perhaps worth noting that before the NHS was established, many health service facilities were run by similar social enterprise-type organisations. Indeed, it was their diversity and unevenness that eventually led to the NHS being conceived. In particular, the extremes in quality and coverage and the lack of equitable access became intolerable. So, while diversity may be valued as an end in itself, and because it can result in services tailored to local needs and preferences, an issue for policy makers is how much diversity can be tolerated before it is deemed problematic and unacceptable. Such issues arise in the matter of priority setting or in rationing health care, with charges of 'postcode prescribing' or the 'postcode lottery' giving rise to concern (see Chapter Five).

Intra-UK health system divergence

Wales and Scotland, as noted above, have resisted going down the market route and in Scotland's case never more so than under its current government, led by the Scottish Nationalists. Successive Scottish governments have adopted the theme of integration and partnership to distinguish its direction, while in Wales, the importance of voice rather than choice in public services has been emphasised. Both countries have been at pains to stress the importance of partnerships and of working collectively with all stakeholders in preference to separating purchasers or commissioners from providers.

As has already been noted, a feature of post-devolution UK health policy has been the growing divergence of arrangements within each of the four countries making up the UK. There were always administrative and organisational differences prior to political devolution, since health care was already a devolved responsibility in administrative terms (Hunter and Wistow 1987; Hunter and Williamson 1991). But political devolution has given a new impetus to greater diversity (Hunter 2007). Although still in its infancy with a long way to go before demonstrating its distinctiveness, devolution has already given rise to several instances of substantive policy differences between the four countries. These are most notable in Scotland and Wales, in particular in Scotland, where the government enjoys greater powers than the Welsh Assembly Government as a result of the Scottish devolution settlement, although the settlement in Wales is under review and is likely to lead to further devolution. The devolution settlement in Scotland is also subject to further devolved powers as a result of the SNP's 2015 election victory.

In Scotland, prescription charges have been abolished and social care is free. Scotland was also the first country in the UK to introduce a ban on smoking in public places – over a year ahead of England. The NHS also has a different structure in Scotland and has not been subjected to the permanent revolution that has been inflicted on its English counterpart in recent years. The Scottish system is altogether more integrated and akin to the structure that existed in England and Wales prior to the experiment with an internal market introduced by the last Conservative government in the early 1990s. There is no longer a purchaser–provider separation in Scotland, and foundation hospital trusts, which were introduced into England and enjoy a degree of independence from central control denied other health care bodies, have no equivalent in Scotland (or Wales for that matter). Hospitals and primary care services come under the overall control of 14 health boards in Scotland.

In Wales, too, there is an integrated structure, with much greater emphasis on joint working between local government and the health service. However, although Wales, like Scotland, has escaped much of the upheaval occurring in England, it is about to go through a period of turbulence as smaller authorities are merged into larger entities. But the emphasis on a top-down, target-driven approach to achieving health care objectives has so far been absent from Wales and Scotland, where a less punitive, more partnership-oriented approach is favoured. Indeed, the Kerr report adopted a set of 'C' words to describe the future direction of the NHS in Scotland, different from those used in England. Eschewing notions of choice and competition, as favoured in England, collaboration and collectivism were chosen as constituting the core values of the Scottish health system.

However, the substantive difference between the respective reform strategies may not be as great as first appearances suggest. In considering the role and meaning of values in the Scottish health service and comparing and contrasting developments between England and Scotland, Kerr and Feeley note that:

> at their extremes, in England, competition to improve standards could lead to fragmentation, whereas in Scotland, increased collectivism could lead to stagnation. The true outcome is likely to sit somewhere closer to the median for both approaches; on the one hand, the health service is so interdependent that fragmentation would be limited, and on the other, why shouldn't collaborative networks compete with each other? (Kerr and Feeley 2007: 34)

Or might the differences be regarded as significant? In another passage, Kerr and Feeley, observing that there are two health care systems (one in Scotland and one in England) that have started from the same place in so far as their founding values are concerned, insist that the two systems 'have moved in significantly different directions, both in terms of the coding of those values into policies and in terms of how those values have been adapted and revealed in the process of making policy' (2007: 34). While both health systems acknowledge that the status quo is not an option, 'there is a dispute that the only answer to the "intractable inefficiencies" of the NHS is for a market-based relationship between hospital and patient' (Kerr and Feeley 2007: 35). It is too early yet to tell which approach is likely to deliver the most health gain.

Apart from differences in the structure and organisation of the Scottish and English health systems, policy differences are also evident between Wales and Scotland on the one hand and England on the other, although it is more difficult to pinpoint exactly how significant these are or will prove to be. Separating the rhetoric from the reality remains an important task for the policy analyst and commentator. At the same time, there is some optimism that the smaller size of the devolved polities, together with the commitment of their respective governments to find different solutions to problems that have eluded their predecessors, will give rise to experimentation and a determination not to ride on the coat-tails of the English.

With the arrival in Scotland in May 2010 of a government led by the Scottish National Party (SNP), which achieved an impressive victory via a prevailing electoral system designed to prevent one-party dominance, greater divergence has occurred. In many ways this is natural, since devolution seems pointless if the potential for greater diversity is not exploited. On the other hand, powerful pressures exist to conform to the policy context determined by England, especially given its size and the existence of a large number of think tanks and analysts all actively generating new ideas and solutions (Laffin 2007; Smith et al 2008). In this regard, size does matter. On the other hand, following the Scottish independence referendum in September 2014 and the impressive political gains made by the SNP in the 2015 general election, such developments make it more likely that Scotland will secure significantly greater devolved powers than previously and chart a distinctive way forward in which public service remains a high priority.

Hitherto, the countries outside England have resisted the tough target regime established there, as well as the emphasis on choice and competition. But Scotland and Wales have not escaped strong pressure from England to emulate the 'success' of English policies, with the NHS in Wales in particular coming under relentless attack from the UK government for failing to adopt similar policies. This is despite a comparison of the four health systems showing little evidence that market reforms have had any appreciable effect on the NHS's performance in England (Bevan et al 2014). Indeed, based on trends over time from the late 1990s to 2011/12 or 2012/13 where data were available, the report revealed that performance had improved in all three countries. The authors concluded that overall their research 'suggests that despite hotly contested policy differences between the UK health systems since devolution on structure, competition, patient choice and the use of non-NHS providers, there is no evidence linking these policy differences to a matching divergence of performance, at least on the measures available across the four UK countries' (Bevan et al 2014: 2).

Conclusion

This chapter has described and reviewed the critiques of the health system reform strategies pursued by successive governments since the late 1990s and has shown where there has been continuity and divergence. The focus on markets, choice and competition in England has been a consistent feature of the reform strategy, although within this overall thrust there have been various policy developments that do not immediately cohere. A renewed emphasis on integrated care is a case in point. The absence of policy coherence has been a source of considerable frustration among health care staff as well as confusing to outsiders, whether patients, clients or members of the public.

As was noted in Chapter One, there exists no convincing evidence base to support any of the assertions underpinning the reform types depicted by Stevens or others who have offered similar schema (see, for example, Le Grand 2007). Despite their claim to be a pragmatic response to the realities of delivering health care, and despite the highly selective use of evidence in their support, these assertions have been informed more by ideology and values, which may well explain why successive reforms of health systems have followed a cyclical pattern, moving from bureaucratic reforms to market reforms, much in the manner suggested by Alford and described in Chapter One.

What has also become much more notable in the UK over the past few years has been the impact on the NHS of political devolution within the UK. There are now four different health systems operating in the UK, albeit with the same overall set of values, although even here there may be some different nuances emerging. Moreover, with some notable exceptions, it is not clear how far the differences will go in substantive terms or whether choice and competition that hold such a tight and powerful grip on health policy in England will not also feature in some form in other parts of the UK in time.

It would have been possible, and certainly more plausible in the light of successive governments' own diagnosis of the problems, to chart an alternative reform scenario that took into account the special nature of professional work in the context of a complex public service that required to be understood in its own terms rather than as something to be hollowed out and rendered fit for an inappropriate business model. Many of these ideas, as Webster has pointed out, took the NHS 'a long way from the founding principles that the government is pledged to uphold' (2002: 258). We return to what such an alternative scenario might look like in the final chapter and assess its likely chances of success.

FIVE

Priority setting in health systems

Introduction

A recurring policy dilemma for health systems concerns the rationing of health care, or, as some prefer to call it, priority setting. The discourse here is about the extent to which rationing health care should (or can) be explicit or whether the implications of this are too painful to contemplate, which makes implicit rationing a more attractive option. This chapter reviews the arguments on both sides. These continue to preoccupy commentators. Taking issue with Mechanic's (1995) argument that explicit approaches to rationing are 'too damaging to public and patient trust in services', and one with which this author has much sympathy (Hunter 1997), Williams and colleagues are convinced that implicit rationing is both 'ethically and politically unacceptable.' They proceed from the assumption that 'explicit priority setting is a legitimate and necessary feature of contemporary policy and practice in health care' (Williams et al 2012: 125). For their part, Light and Hughes consider that critics of explicit rationing make important points about the limitations of formal attempts at rationing but that implicit rationing can cover up poor professional practice and quality of care. They favour a solution that 'lies in re-conceptualising professionalism around accountability rather than autonomy', thereby ensuring that 'the use of power in both explicit and implicit rationing are subject to transparent review' (Light and Hughes 2002: 12). They also make a plea for a sociological perspective to counter-balance and challenge the dominant economic view with its tendency to frame the issues 'in a narrow and misleading way' (Light and Hughes 2002: 17) and 'set up an over-blunt dichotomy between treatment and denial, when what is at issue is more nuanced and uncertain' (Light and Hughes 2002: 15).

Back in the1980s and 1990s, the term 'rationing' was on the lips of every health policy maker in countries around the world, including in the US, New Zealand and the UK. The word was often invoked as a term of abuse with pejorative overtones and as demonstrating a serious deficiency in respect of health policy and the evident inability of governments to make available sufficient resources to enable legitimate health care needs to be met appropriately. Passionate debates were rife over developments such as so-called postcode prescribing or the postcode lottery, whereby patients' access to health care depends on where they live. As Tudor Hart's 'inverse care law' put it, the actual need for care seemed to have little to do with what was often prescribed, or not, as the case may be (Tudor Hart 1971). The paradox in the UK of a national health service that seems anything but national upon closer inspection has provided the media with ample scare stories of often-vulnerable people being denied treatments that are available in another part of the country. Since devolution to Scotland and Wales in the late 1990s, stories abound of people crossing the border and receiving treatments not available to them at home. And with the abolition of prescription charges in Wales and moves to phase them out in Scotland, the potential for differential rationing across Britain could be considerable, although it has not so far taken off in such a way as to arouse public concern.

The celebrated Child B case that held the nation's attention in 1995 following legal action brought against a local health authority in England by the child's father for refusing to spend £75,000 on further treatment for his daughter encapsulated all the emotional, political, economic and other issues that arise in decisions about who, and who not, to treat. It was a classic example of health care rationing *in extremis* and it polarised both professional and public opinion, with some supporting the health authority's decision while others sided with the father in his attempt to do all he could to extend his daughter's life.

A couple of decades or so later, there seems to be less heated discussion about rationing. The dreaded 'r' word is now rarely used, although that may be about to change as a consequence of the severe pressure on NHS finances following the government's austerity policies to tackle the fiscal deficit and the squeeze on public spending. These are beginning to cause problems in the delivery of care on the front line, despite the government's insistence that spending on health has been protected. This may be true, but it is occurring against a backdrop of a growing and ageing population. Therefore, 'despite its relative protection, the NHS is showing increasing signs of financial distress' (Charlesworth 2015: 5). These signs have manifested themselves in various ways. For example, 81% of all NHS acute hospitals in England were in deficit at the end of September 2014, and six out of 10 NHS providers (acute hospitals, community services and mental health trusts) could not balance their books halfway through 2014–15. The explanation for rationing being largely off the political agenda may be because up until 2008 significant new money flowed into the NHS and displaced rationing as a central policy concern (Klein 2007). Whatever the explanation, the terms currently in vogue are 'choice' and 'priority setting'. The era of the rational rationers seems to be a thing of the past, apart from a few forlorn economists who continue to press for a proper public debate about what a publicly funded health system can or should afford. The arguments for rationing are likely to resurface as a result of the pressures on public finances, including health. But when politicians do pick up the argument, they usually come to regret it. An example of this is when the former health secretary, Patricia Hewitt, overruled the National Institute for Health and Clinical Excellence (NICE) – the body charged with assessing the cost-effectiveness of new treatments – and allowed the cancer drug Herceptin to be made available to all those who might benefit from it.

As was noted in the last chapter, politicians all too readily ignore the lessons from history. In 2010, for instance, David Cameron set up the Cancer Drugs Fund with a budget of £200 million, in order to deliver his promise to make available to cancer patients expensive drugs rejected by NICE for use in the NHS because of their high cost and limited effectiveness. These drugs can offer relief and an improved quality of care, but only over a period of a few months. Nevertheless, as a political move it proved popular, although not without controversy. Some patient groups believe that the pharmaceutical companies manufacturing these expensive drugs are over-charging for them as a result of the Cancer Drugs Fund having been introduced, while others believe they are the victims of discrimination and query why cancer should be accorded special treatment over other life-threatening conditions. As a result, not only has the fund exceeded its budget limit, but it has raised serious issues about the government's whole approach to priority setting and where it leaves NICE, the body officially charged with the task.

Indeed, the Cancer Drugs Fund has undermined NICE in overturning its recommendations and acting as a parallel rationing body (Rid et al 2015). The current NHS chief executive has made it clear that this is not sustainable, and advocates a return to the status quo, with sole responsibility for drug assessment remaining with NICE. NHS England's strategy document, *The National Health Service Five Year Forward View*, states: 'we expect over the next year to consult on a new approach to converging its assessment and prioritisation processes with a revised approach from NICE' (NHS England 2014: 34). At the same time, it is accepted that changes in NICE's methods and approach may be required to reflect current concerns and pressures on health care, including greater awareness of patient views and expectations.

A case in point concerns NICE's revised policy regarding the use of statins as a preventive measure, with GPs receiving a payment for prescribing the cholesterol-lowering drugs under the quality and outcomes framework arrangement. The recommendation is that statins be prescribed for people with a 10% risk of developing a serious cardiovascular condition over 10 years. 'Statins work, they are very cheap, and are becoming considerably cheaper as they come off patent which in a cost limited health service is a big consideration to think about' (NICE 2014). This policy may result in mass medication of the population, despite most healthy people in receipt of statins not succumbing to any life-threatening condition. The danger of medicalising the population in this way has triggered ethical concerns and a view, especially evident among many GPs, that NICE has both exceeded its remit and perhaps shown bias, capitulating to pressures from the pharmaceutical industry, which stands to gain from increasing the number of people using medications (Greenhalgh et al 2014). Questions have also been raised about the long-term side effects of statins and a belief that for some people these can be serious. The issue is not so much that NICE may be wrong, but that patients may prefer to avoid taking statins every day for the rest of their lives if not actually required to in response to a diagnosed problem, and instead adopt a healthier lifestyle. The concern is that this option is less likely to be offered if GPs are incentivised to prescribe statins.

Approaches to rationing health care

Although priority setting and rationing may be regarded as essentially the same activity, the former term is preferred by policy makers since it does not carry the pejorative overtones of denial often associated with the term 'rationing'. Whereas priority setting is about deciding what the NHS should provide, rationing is about deciding what the NHS should not provide, or to whom treatment should be denied (BMA 1995). To suggest explicitly that something is being denied someone is anathema to politicians who feel obliged to give the public the reassurance that everything is available to everyone in order to meet their needs. But whatever term is used, in practice a range of mechanisms to ration health care have been identified as being in common use. Known as the 'five Ds', they are set out in Box 5.1.

Box 5.1: Rationing mechanisms

Deterrence. Rationing can occur by obstructing the demands for health care through mechanisms such as user co-payments (eg prescription and dental charges) or the inconvenient location of services and facilities, which cuts down on their use.

Delay. Waiting lists (and times) are a good example of delay functioning as a holding area (and often for sound clinical reasons) to buffer excess demand.

Deflection. GPs may act as gatekeepers to secondary care to deflect demand for secondary care and channel it into primary care; or GPs may choose to deflect demand for health services altogether by shifting it to social services and therefore onto another agency's budget – a tactic also known as 'cost shunting'. Giving patients more information about treatments, outcomes and side effects may also have this result as people may choose not to proceed to visit their GP or hospital – the purpose of NHS Direct is in part to deflect pressure on the services by acting a filter or gatekeeper to GPs.

Dilution. Demand for care can be diluted by reducing the amount of service offered, (eg the use of fewer tests or attendances). Clinical freedom may also serve as a means of dilution whereby decisions not to treat are couched in terms of clinical decisions, thus obscuring what may actually be rationing decisions.

Denial. The exclusion of services from the NHS or their denial to individual patients or groups of patients (eg in-vitro fertilisation (IVF) services, tattoo removal).

Source: Harrison and Hunter (1994: 25–30).

Given the pressures evident in funding the UK NHS, it seems premature to claim that the issue of rationing health care been successfully resolved. For a time this was the case, largely as a result of an injection of new money into health care services. The advent of NICE, a widely respected organisation that is the envy of many other countries keen to have a similar regulatory body, has also been a significant factor and remains so, although the context in which NICE is now operating and will operate in the future is very different from when it was created. It is certainly the case that under NICE, health care rationing has been successfully managed in a way that has largely retained public support. But like all the policy cleavages considered in this book, nothing is permanent and many of the issues that might have been thought to have been resolved have a nasty knack of resurfacing in the same or a familiar guise.

Whatever the reasons for rationing having lost its high profile and emotional pulling power over the past couple of decades or so, health care systems that are publicly financed still have to make choices over what can and cannot be covered. Most countries face high demands and have limited resources with which to meet them, and many have struggled to devise mechanisms that will fairly allocate available resources between competing demands.

The view adopted in this chapter is that significant resources are already being invested in health services – especially in the years between 2002 and 2008 in the UK, with the level of investment (9.4% of GDP) approaching the average level of spend in the EU – and that there is in any case never a right level of spending. Unless it can be claimed that existing investment in health care is always appropriate and is never spent on activities or interventions that are, knowingly or unknowingly, ineffective (and therefore wasteful of limited resources that could be better spent on interventions of proven efficacy), a necessary prerequisite must be to ensure that current or proposed interventions are as far as possible evidence-based. This is certainly the view adopted by those who are critical of economists and others who believe that rationing is inevitable and unavoidable (Hunter 1997).

Some of the various mechanisms for making choices in health care, in addition to those listed in Box 5.1, are reviewed later in this chapter. But it is important to note at the outset that none is perfect or provides the complete answer to the difficult dilemma of choosing how, and on what, to spend finite health resources. Indeed, the provision of health and health care are imperfect activities, which is what makes them such intensely political concerns. There is no perfect or rational solution to matters of priority setting or what has become known, somewhat pejoratively, as rationing.

Even NICE, which has commendably approached its work in the most dispassionate and scientifically evidence-based way possible despite inhabiting an intensely political environment, has been forced to review some of its decisions in the light of a public outcry about the merits of its judgements. The issue then arises of whose evidence is important in reaching a decision of whether or not to approve a particular treatment. Is it the view of the expert or that of the patient or user that should prevail? To its credit, NICE has managed fairly successfully over a long period to steer a steady course in this often tricky territory. Indeed, the environment within which it operates can only get more treacherous as government policies to promote patient choice and the notion of consumerism in health care raise expectations of what patients think they should be entitled to (see Chapter Six). The NHS Constitution, which establishes the principles and values of the NHS in England and sets out the rights to which patients public and staff are entitled and the responsibilities to which these groups owe to one another to ensure that the NHS operates fairly and effectively, can only fuel such expectations further. All this is happening against a backdrop of often fierce disagreement among experts on what interventions are appropriate for particular conditions. For example, there are those who subscribe to surgical and pharmaceutical solutions in order to tackle obesity, especially among children. Others, however, regard the issue as being a societal and structural one, with individuals at the mercy of the food industry and producers, and of market-led policies that are insufficiently regulated. They conclude that the appropriate policy response has to be one that addresses such structural determinants and that to focus on, or 'blame', the individual is misplaced and offers no lasting solution.

For a government anxious to be seen to be doing something and to making a visible difference, does the answer lie in putting resources into new drugs and surgical specialties that deal with the symptoms of a complex problem such as obesity? Does it lie in dispensing lifestyle advice on diet and exercise? Or does it lie in going upstream and tackling the source of the problem, which resides in a combination of food production, environmental planning, sedentary lifestyles and so on? Even if there is to be a balance of investment across the range of policy options, from individual lifestyles to structural determinants, deciding what this optimal mix should be is an immensely complex issue, especially when most governments are poor at looking at problems and their solutions in a holistic, joined-up way. Scotland, under its former Chief Medical Officer, Sir Harry Burns, has attempted to introduce a whole of government and whole of society approach to deep-seated public health problems, but it is too early to be sure if this new approach is working (Burns 2015).

Given the enormity and complexity of the challenge, most governments tend to duck or fudge the issues and fail to offer inspired leadership. Moreover, many pursue policies that themselves are often internally contradictory and send mixed messages about what the true direction of policy is. For instance, encouraging choice and local diversity may be entirely legitimate ends in themselves. But if they result in greater inequity among those seeking support and care, or if they lead to widely varying levels of care and treatment in different parts of the country, can this be tolerated in countries that operate national health services and have a history of centralised policy making? In the UK, for example, these dilemmas have swung back and forth over the years. At one time, the answer was seen to lie in greater transparency and consistency across the country. So, for example, the introduction of national service frameworks for conditions like diabetes, coronary heart disease, mental health and so on was seen as reinstating a form of central planning, offering a standardised approach to policy and to appropriate interventions for uniform implementation across the country. But, on other occasions, as in the 2000s, the answer was seen to lie in the individual and the locally made decisions of bodies such as primary care trusts (PCTs), which spent the bulk (around 80%) of resources available for health and health care. But if a PCT, or its successor, the clinical commissioning group (CCG), decided against prescribing a particular drug that a neighbouring PCT or CCG might agree to fund, there is likely to be a media uproar about unfairness and lack of consistency. In a country, such as the UK, that is densely populated and has strong national media, it becomes politically very difficult to balance such central and local pressures and steer a way forward that is acceptable to everyone.

And yet, in 2015, renewed enthusiasm for devolution and for giving local government new powers and increased responsibilities for health is evident among politicians. Initiatives such as DevoManc (part of what is known as the Northern Powerhouse experiment) and new powers for the major cities are being seized upon as the solution to an over-centralised state. The proposals for devolution are also a response to concerns that if countries like Scotland and Wales can have devolved powers what about England which is the largest country making up the UK? How an issue like rationing will fare under a devolved polity and what the implications are for the recommendations of a national body like NICE remain to be seen, but it is worth noting that the creation of the NHS was itself partly a response to the patchwork nature and uneven quality of health services originally run by local authorities and voluntary bodies. For some commentators, the solution seems to lie in a national public debate on what health services will, and will not, cover. Economists in particular have argued *ad nauseam* for such a rational approach to rationing. However, others consider that such a debate is a wholly unrealistic proposition and that the issues are simply too complex and dynamic to be resolved through such means. They maintain that all that can be hoped for is not that the 'muddling through' approach is abandoned, but that it can be managed in an improved manner – what has been termed 'muddling through elegantly' (Hunter 1997).

In practice, and being realistic, rationing will always be an imperfect and contested activity where explicit decisions may not always be the best way forward and where a degree of implicitness, or muddling through, may offer the optimal approach, even if is difficult openly to acknowledge this. But, as was noted earlier, this need not mean that clinicians making those decisions, whether implicit or explicit, are not held to account for them. They need to be accountable since there cannot be a reliance on trust alone. Different countries have adopted different approaches and policy responses to the dilemma of rationing health care. These range from excluding those procedures for which there is insufficient evidence of cost-effectiveness (as in the

UK through the work of NICE and its equivalent in Scotland, the Scottish Intercollegiate Guidelines Network [SIGN]), to developing clinical scoring systems to establish health priorities, to defining essential core services that receive funding (as in New Zealand) or a basic insurance package (as in the Netherlands), to ranking treatments as a basis for funding decisions (as in the case of the exercise undertaken in the state of Oregon in the US). Details of these and similar schemes can be found in edited volumes by Coulter and Ham (2000) and Ham and Robert (2003) and will not be described further here. Any attempt to circumscribe health care and establish the criteria for core services, thereby identifying both entitlements and exclusions, is highly contestable. In practice, excluded services have tended to creep in by the back door (Klein 2007).

In its analysis of how best to accommodate competing demands within a constrained budget, the British Medical Association (BMA 2007) wants to see more scope for local health economies to determine how best to use their budgets within a set of nationally determined core services. The problem with this proposal is that identified earlier: when does local discretion become postcode rationing? If central prescription is at odds with local priorities – as in the case of some NICE recommendations – which of those priorities should prevail, and who decides? There are no easy answers to such tricky policy concerns.

The National Institute for Health and Care Excellence

The UK approach to rationing has been to avoid any attempt at an explicit ranking of treatments, or identifying a set of core services or basic basket of services despite calls for these from some quarters. Rationing has for the most part been left to local decision and discretion, with national policy makers for the most part staying well clear from such a politically hot topic. On the rare occasions, usually concerning high-profile drugs, when politicians have strayed into the treacherous waters surrounding rationing – as former health secretary Hewitt did over Herceptin, mentioned earlier, or as Frank Dobson earlier did over Viagra when it first came onto the market – they have always found the experience a bruising one, albeit never admitting as much (see further below). A similar fate seems likely to befall the Cancer Drugs Fund. The Fund was established by the coalition government in 2011 to permit access to expensive cancer drugs that NICE had not approved. Its budget was set at £200 million in 2013/14, increased to £340 million in 2014/15 but is estimated to rise to £410 million this year which amounts to a 70% overspend. Controlling the rising cost of the Fund is a priority for NHS England. There are also moves to bring the Fund more into line with NICE's working practices. Many economists and other observers consider the Fund to be a waste of money as well as undermining NICE (Klaxton 2015).

However, these skirmishes as well as the experience of the Cancer Drugs Fund have served the useful purpose of convincing ministers that rationing is a no-win issue for them and that a different approach, one that is as far as possible evidence-based, is preferable. They therefore now tend to approach rationing from a different perspective altogether, taking the view that it makes no sense explicitly to ration health care when it is known that many existing treatments and procedures are of doubtful efficacy and should be discontinued before any attempt at explicit rationing is sanctioned. The argument is that it would be morally indefensible to ration care prior to ensuring that all current services provided are evidence-based and effective. Hence the creation in 1999 of the National Institute for Clinical Excellence, known as NICE, which covers the NHS in England and Wales (Rawlins 2015).

NICE is charged with assessing the evidence base for particular interventions and with providing cost-effective guidance to the NHS. It provides guidance both in terms of individual health technologies (such as medicines, medical devices, diagnostic techniques and procedures) and the clinical management of specific conditions. It provides three main types of guidance:

- technology appraisals of new and existing health technologies;
- clinical guidelines and protocols for the management of specific diseases and conditions;
- safety and efficacy decisions about new interventions.

NICE's advice is intended to end postcode prescribing and to challenge the persistence of what are regarded as unacceptable variations in the quality of care within an ostensibly national health service. To this end, NICE is concerned not only with producing guidance on what is effective but also with how implementation can be effected to secure actual changes in practice. Local health organisations are expected to adopt NICE guidance when determining local priorities and making resource allocation decisions, although they may also decide to act differently in meeting the health care needs of their patients. However, in 1999 the High Court ruled that NICE guidance could not be legally binding. The judgment concerned a case where the drug manufacturer Pfizer contested a circular issued by the then health secretary Frank Dobson following advice from NICE and asking GPs not to prescribe Viagra. The High Court ruled that the circular was unlawful in preventing doctors from exercising their clinical judgement. As a result, NICE guidance cannot replace the knowledge and skills of local PCTs or frontline professionals, although practitioners would need to have good reasons for not following the guidance.

Implementing NICE guidance has always been an area of weakness and remains so. As NICE's chief executive, Andrew Dillon, has stated, 'there is little point in us developing guidance if no one puts it into practice' (Dillon 2007). In response to this situation, NICE has established a dedicated team to support those working in local NHS organisations. A full complement of implementation support tools is available and accompanies each piece of guidance issued. In response to perceived weaknesses in the commissioning function as noted in Chapter Three, NICE has produced a series of commissioning guides. Their aim is to reduce spending on treatments that do not improve patient care or do not represent good value for money. The guides set benchmarks to determine the level of service needed for a particular area. They also offer advice in respect of local needs assessment and opportunities for disinvestment. However, it is well known, and supported by evidence, that the mere provision of information is no guarantee of subsequent action. It is one factor among many in the context of policy change and probably not the most important.

Clinician attitudes, culture, custom and practice, financial stability and so on are all probably more important influences on decision making. Overcoming the barriers to changing practice is also an issue of concern to NICE since its work ultimately has little value unless these issues are understood and confronted. Finally, although the issue of resources is no excuse for not complying with NICE guidance, it remains a fuzzy area, with NHS organisations often complaining of the volume of guidance requiring attention and its associated cost. The annual budget allocation to the NHS includes an allowance for the estimated extra cost of implementing NICE guidance, but this amount is neither ring-fenced nor identified separately in budgets, which may make it easier for the resources to be spent on other activities, such as meeting government-imposed targets.

In April 2005, NICE was renamed the National Institute for Health and Clinical Excellence as a result of a merger with the Health Development Agency that was tasked with developing an evidence base for public health. Responsibility for public health passed to NICE in a move that at the time surprised policy watchers. The marriage was not an obvious one, given NICE's origins and focus on clinical care, and there were concerns that public health would remain in the shadows of its clinical guidelines work. But, largely thanks to the Centre for Public Health Excellence under Mike Kelly's leadership, NICE earned the respect of the public health community for its public health guidance, much of which addressed the main policy challenges in respect of alcohol misuse, obesity, physical exercise, mental health and so on and began to make its mark (Kelly 2007). Apart from its public health work, NICE as a whole remained firmly focused on the NHS and on secondary health care until 2013, when the coalition government decided it should include social care in its brief. So, while still retaining its acronym, NICE became known as the National Institute for Health and Care Excellence.

Such a move means that NICE now embraces virtually the whole care pathway from first contact with health care through to social care and care in the community. The move has also come at a time when the government is encouraging closer integration between health and social care through the Better Care Fund. With Mike Kelly's retirement in 2015, it was decided that the Centre for Public Health Excellence should merge with social care to form a division of health and social care within NICE. Critics of the move claim that the changes, and in particular the loss of Kelly, undermine the importance and profile of public health within NICE. Time will tell if the critics are right. However, since a major part of NICE's guidance work now concerns activities located with local government, NICE is having to face a new and different audience and one that continues to view NICE as an NHS body concerned with clinical care. Becoming as familiar a presence in local government as in the NHS represents a major challenge for NICE in future.

Rational rationing: the limits to economic approaches

Economic techniques to assist with priority setting have been developed over the years, notable among these being cost-effectiveness analysis, quality-adjusted life years and programme budgeting and marginal analysis. However, despite the best endeavours of economists and those promoting their cause, economic approaches to priority setting have had only limited impact in practice (Goddard et al 2006). It is not hard to see why rational rationing has failed to secure wide or lasting political support. This is largely because of the existence of different types of rationality, of which that proffered by economists is but one and not always, if ever, that preferred by policy makers.

As Goddard and colleagues rightly acknowledge:

> [I]t is not necessarily methodological shortcomings that are the main reason for lack of impact, but rather the wider context of public-sector decision making. From this viewpoint, although economic evaluation offers one approach to setting priorities, it may be equally rational for decision makers to behave in different ways, depending on

the context in which decision making takes place. (Goddard
et al 2006: 81)

The authors argue that models of political economy may have more
to offer in an attempt to understand why decision makers diverge
from economic rationality when setting priorities in health. Of
course, for political scientists, the notion of competing rationalities
and the broader political, institutional and environmental constraints
operating on decision makers come as no surprise. But for economists
such as Goddard and colleagues, this way of viewing decisions and
understanding how they have been arrived at is clearly a revelation,
which probably says a lot about the state of economics and the narrow,
mechanistic view of human behaviour underpinning economic models.

An exception is McDonald's (2002) study of how the 'rational'
approach underpinning health economic analyses could be reconciled
with the author's earlier experiences of real-world NHS decision
making as an accountant before she became a health economist. In
her studies at York University, she was critical of the 'failure of health
economists to engage with real world decision-makers' and with the
teaching of health economics largely 'in a political vacuum' (McDonald
2002: 2). She searched in vain for published work relating to the use
of health economics in practice. Her two-year research study took the
form of study of decision making in the health authority in which she
was employed as a health economist.

The picture of decision making that emerged from the research
proved far removed from the prescriptions of the rational model
to which health economists seem wedded, even if only as an ideal
type. However, such a model is not especially helpful in furthering
understanding of how decisions are made and therefore of how
priorities are chosen. McDonald identified a number of features of
real-world decision making in which decision makers:

- are forced to pursue many objectives simultaneously
- do not always share common objectives

- are not trying to maximise anything and may be unwilling to be explicit about their goals
- are reactive and problem-definition fluid in their decision-making (McDonald 2002: 155–7)

Furthermore, McDonald found that:

- action is less a means to an end than an end in itself
- more is always better than less
- the views and values of decision-makers exist prior to problem-definition and 'rational' optional appraisal processes
- ambiguity is a central feature of decision-making
- policy actors enjoy wide discretion and freedom from central control, yet perceive themselves as powerless
- knowledge is contingent and subjective. (McDonald: 157–63)

Of course, students of policy analysis like Lipsky (1980) will not be surprised at such findings. What may be more surprising is the persistence among economists and policy makers that 'rational' decision making is somehow possible if only the impediments to perfect implementation could be resolved and/or removed. That these impediments are often rooted in power relations and political beliefs about how best to provide care in a given situation seems to have escaped health economists, or certainly those of a neoclassical persuasion who have yet to be convinced of the value of 'alternative' economics known as the behavioural economics approach.

McDonald's research confirms the unwillingness and inability of managers and clinicians 'to engage in the sort of systematic and explicit decision-making processes which lie at the heart of health economics' (2002: 164). But their reasons for rejecting such processes are entirely rational since the coping mechanisms adopted enable the system to survive and deliver. McDonald suggests that to ignore such a reality and seek to impose rational approaches would put in jeopardy the system's 'life support' apparatus, thereby demonstrating that 'the pursuit of rationality is itself irrational' (2002: 166).

In their study of rationing in health care, Williams and colleagues (2012) acknowledge that more attention needs to be paid to the implementation of priority-setting decisions in messy, complex systems that are often intensely political. For this reason, they argue in favour of connecting priority setting to the broader literature on change, innovation and improvement in health care. This perspective also had to include notions of leadership and being able to lead with political astuteness.

For McDonald and other observers of complex systems such as the NHS, or, indeed, any health system anywhere in the world, 'the existence of multiple and competing goals which are not amenable to explicit prioritisation' is a given (McDonald 2002: 169). Such multiple and conflicting goals remain much in evidence in the current NHS. For example, postcode prescribing is deemed unacceptable yet at the same time devolved decision making and what has been termed 'the new localism' are being actively promoted. Then there is the work of NICE and its endorsement of a new treatment that NHS organisations are obliged to provide in appropriate cases. If explicit rationing is outlawed but, at the same time, additional resources are not forthcoming, what are beleaguered NHS bodies to do except fall back on the coping strategies and adaptive mechanisms that permit them to manage uncertainty and ambiguity?

Where values conflict, there is little point in urging decision makers to adopt 'rational' methods to aid their decisions. As is the case with the other policy cleavages, or health debates that are the subject of this book, the issues have less to do with the absence of rational methods and decision rules than with power and puzzlement. *Pace* Heclo (1975), some dilemmas in health policy may simply be too difficult and 'unwinnable' (see also Hunter 1980).

Involving the public in priority setting

It is politically popular to involve the public in priority setting or rationing, or, indeed, in any other aspect of health policy. To appear to be doing otherwise in the 21st century amounts to political suicide. We live in an age where politicians are expected to follow public opinion rather than to lead it. Views like Loughlin's (1996), suggesting that there must be a query over how rational rationing can be when society may not in fact be rational, are clearly not in fashion.

In a market system, such dilemmas do not arise since a health system that is reliant upon market mechanisms like choice and competition for delivering health care in effect delegates the priority-setting problem to the 'hidden hand' of the marketplace without recourse to conscious, probably flawed, policy making (Goddard et al 2006). However, such systems pose other problems: in particular, so it is claimed, the fact that consumers tend to choose the most expensive procedure that they can afford in the belief that the most costly will also be the best (Torgerson and Gosden 2000). This tendency may explain in part why the US spends a much greater proportion of its GNP on health care compared with other less market-oriented health systems. Not only are consumers inclined to choose the most expensive procedure or treatment, but their actions may also result in access to treatments that are no more effective than cheaper alternatives.

Torgerson and Gosden's argument is that by removing health care purchasing decisions from consumers, the NHS model of health care improves efficiency as it allows those with sufficient expertise (doctors) to purchase effective treatments on behalf of patients. Of course, such an approach has been criticised for being paternalistic and for failing to acknowledge the flaws in allowing a group of experts unchallenged authority over an individual's life. Moreover, the NHS lacks adequate accountability to the public, since the agencies entrusted with decision making and resource allocation powers are appointed and not directly elected. Indirect accountability through the electoral system is a poor substitute, since people rarely cast their votes on the basis of a single issue. However, these difficulties only go to demonstrate that, as Torgerson and Gosden put it, 'rationing is painful, complicated, and difficult' (2000: 1679). We know, they assert, from numerous public opinion surveys that smokers, drug users, heavy drinkers and older people should receive lower priority than others. Experiments with citizens' juries conducted by the Institute for Public Policy Research (IPPR) in 1996 suggest that, with proper investment in witness evidence and the opportunity for issues to be explained, members of juries will arrive at different judgements and preferences from those assumed or asserted at the outset (Lenaghan 1996). Summarising the five pilots run by the IPPR, Lenaghan concluded that citizens' juries as a form of public involvement offered citizens 'an opportunity to consider and discuss policy issues in sufficient detail to reach a sophisticated understanding of the issues' (1996: 91). Jurors demonstrated 'a capacity to follow a steep learning curve, skills in cross examining witnesses, willingness to discuss and debate the issues with each other …' (Lenaghan 1996: 91).

Citizens' juries are expensive in terms of resources and time and are not a wholesale solution to the problem of determining who should ration or set priorities. But what they do show is that public opinion may not always be predictable when it comes to health care priorities and that an exclusive focus on hospitals or beds may not always be apparent. As research undertaken by the National Consumer Council has shown, the public's highest priority for funding after beds and staffing was health promotion and helping people to help themselves (National Consumer Council 1998). Also, from their survey work, Ford and Cooke (2000) show that the public support the principle of equity, of equal treatment for older people, and a view that cause of illness is no basis for limiting treatment.

Nevertheless, the challenge of how most effectively to engage the public in setting priorities remains. At a national level, it has been suggested that citizens' juries or a people's assembly might be established to discuss, debate and come to a conclusion about the trade-offs necessary when it comes to the existence of a postcode lottery or the adoption of new treatments. But such devices only work if they are seen to be genuine and credible and able to exert real influence on decision making. If they are seen as 'engagement camouflage' for decisions already taken elsewhere, they will quickly become discredited (Lawson 2007).

Perhaps the answer lies in strengthening an institution such as NICE, which already enjoys a substantial degree of public legitimacy through its Citizens Council that could be enhanced. NICE has demonstrated an ability to be a learning organisation and has been prepared to adapt and change as circumstances demand. The Citizens Council is a panel of 30 members of the public drawn from all social groups to contribute to its thinking about how to value health care treatments and their impact. Members meet once a year for two days at a time and serve for up to three years. They provide NICE with a public perspective on a range of moral and ethical issues that NICE takes into account when producing guidance. The questions and topics identified for discussion are wide-ranging and over the years have included the following: what are the societal values that need to be considered when making decisions about trade-offs between equity and efficiency (May 2014)?; what aspects of benefit, cost and need should NICE take into account when developing social care guidelines (January 2013)?; in what circumstances are incentives to promote individual behaviour change an acceptable way of promoting the health of the public (May 2010)? The Council's recommendations and conclusions are published, discussed by the NICE board and, where appropriate, are incorporated into NICE's methodology.

However, there are limits to how far users and communities can be involved in complex decisions and especially in making them responsible for whatever results. Perhaps of most importance, they should not become an excuse for the withdrawal or abnegation of the state from making difficult decisions.

Implicit versus explicit rationing

The debate on rationing has revolved around those who subscribe to a view that it should remain implicit, and those who consider such a lack of transparency unacceptable and who therefore wish to see the process made much more explicit. While explicit rationing may be intellectually irrefutable, and the rational response to adopt in a perfect world, the messy reality is not conducive to the serious adoption of such a position. For instance, as one clinician explains, 'rule-based rationing' – for that is what explicit rationing amounts to – 'is problematic, because the rules can very quickly become unmanageable' (Ubel 2001: 15). The rules can also become subject to 'gaming' by clinicians as they seek to interpret or bend them to benefit their patients or perhaps a few selected ones. Physicians are notoriously adept at circumventing rules. It seems paradoxical, then, that some physicians should insist that politicians make and apply the rules under which doctors would then be required to operate but which they would have no hesitation in flouting if they were not seen to be helpful. But any form of 'gaming' or creative interpretation of rules hardly amounts to the transparent, publicly defensible form of rationing that the hard-nosed rational rationers favour. Indeed, such an attempt at overtness is surely destined to lead to new forms of covertness. How this might offer a fairer or better way than the present admittedly imperfect arrangements is a matter that those who support explicit rationing have singularly failed to articulate.

Explicit rationing can also give rise to two sources of disutility (Coast 1997). First, citizens become involved in the process of denying care to particular groups of individuals, or particular individuals may experience disutility – 'denial disutility'. Second, disutility may arise when individuals are informed explicitly that their care is being rationed – 'deprivation disutility'. Both types of disutility may be distressing, with the consequence that the clinical benefits of explicitness may be less than expected. The point is that the very attempt at explicitness carries its own disutility, which may outweigh any benefit in moving from an implicit to an explicit approach. The openness and honesty of being explicit may prove too great a burden to bear compared with the equivocation associated with being implicit. As an editorial in *The Lancet* put it: 'the cry of pain that accompanies each revelation of explicit service rationing might eventually become too great to endure' (*Lancet* 1995: 63).

Although rationing health care clearly raises many delicate and difficult political and ethical issues that politicians, managers and health care practitioners confront daily, if we are at all honest and realistic then some of these issues will simply not be confronted because they cannot be. In the cut and thrust of politics they will quite simply be fudged. As was noted above, they are in Heclo's term 'unwinnable'. In such a context, a policy response based on muddling through is not only the most likely option to be adopted in practice but also the most realistic and pragmatic especially if it prevents policy stasis or gridlock.

It may be posited that the currently fashionable managerialist notions of user empowerment, explicitness and transparency are disruptive. The desire for constant probing may actually be counter-productive or rapidly in danger of becoming so; tinkering with and subjecting to bureaucratic scrutiny the delicate workings and operating procedures that have evolved over decades to determine how choices in health care are made. 'Far from helping society to function better and in a more mature manner, such forensic behaviour may be creating a set of circumstances in which it becomes ever more difficult to transact the business sensibly in a given policy sphere' (Hunter 1997: 9).

Finding a middle way

Occupying the middle ground between the two extremes of explicit rationing on the one hand and implicit rationing on the other is an approach known as 'accountability for reasonableness' (Daniels 2000). It shares with implicit approaches the view that principles for rationing cannot, or should not, be made explicit ahead of time. However, like explicit approaches, it calls for transparency and openness about reasoning that all can eventually agree is relevant. Daniels believes that accountability for reasonableness makes it possible to educate stakeholders in the substance of deliberations about fair decisions under resource constraints and, in particular, 'facilitates social learning about limits' (2000: 1301). Adoption of an approach centred on accountability for reasonableness ensures that the grounds for decisions are rendered transparent and open to scrutiny and that appeals to such decisions are allowable with procedures in place to permit revisions of decisions in the light of successful challenges to them.

There is much in common between accountability for reasonableness and the notion introduced earlier of 'muddling through elegantly' (Hunter 1997). This offers an approach to the vexing issue of health care rationing that acknowledges the need for a more realistic and nuanced assessment of the complexities involved. If, as many claim, rationing is a multifaceted and multilevelled activity, to which there are no perfect answers to how it should best be conducted, it needs to be approached accordingly. Hence the appeal of a muddling-through approach that, far from being indefensible and defeatist, acknowledges the dynamic, complex and context-specific nature of rationing.

Professional discretion, or what has been termed 'bedside rationing' (Ubel 2001), lies at the heart of muddling through. The notion of muddling through elegantly, far from implying a conservative defence of the status quo, both accepts and fully acknowledges that improvements are necessary in how decisions on priorities are made, especially at a micro level where doctors and patients interact. Patients are entitled to demand fair dealing on the part of professionals, which might best be assured through a system of procedural rights (Coote and Hunter 1996). This might take the form of guidelines about how decisions are made and by whom. The guidelines would not be concerned with rationing health care. Their purpose would be to establish a set of general principles expressing or restating the values and objectives of the particular health care system in question and setting standards for fair and consistent administrative procedures. Such an overarching explicit framework governing decision making would not preclude implicit, or bedside, rationing at a micro level where professional judgement deemed it to be desirable. This is the essence of muddling through elegantly in situations characterised by extreme uncertainty, where information is poor, incomplete and often contested.

Like Daniels' accountability for reasonableness, muddling through elegantly shares elements of both implicit and explicit approaches. At its root is the importance of a 'negotiated order', or co-production of care, between doctor and patient. As mentioned earlier, Light and

Hughes' notion of holding the medical profession to account to ensure that their power and autonomy are exercised appropriately and in a transparent fashion is also relevant and fits with the idea of accountability for reasonableness (Light and Hughes 2002).

Conclusion

While public discussion of rationing health care appears muted when compared with the state of discourse surrounding the issue back in the 1990s, it seems certain that the issue has not gone away or been finally resolved. Rather, politically it has been managed in such a way as to keep it off the policy agenda. But it simmers beneath the surface and occasionally breaks out in a flurry of media scare stories about people suffering and/or dying after they have been denied essential treatment.

But thanks largely to the Labour government's injection of significant new money into the NHS between 2002 and 2008, and the work of NICE set up by the Labour government in 1999, mention of rationing has been rare of late. But all that has begun to change as NHS funding has flatlined at best and seen a reduction at worst as the government's austerity measures start to bite. Whereas spending under Labour saw the highest period of spending growth for the NHS at 8.7% a year in real terms between 2001/02 and 2004/05, the coalition government witnessed the lowest rate of growth in health spending since 1955 (0.6%) (Charlesworth 2015). There is therefore every prospect of rationing rearing its head and breaking the surface.

Few would deny that rationing is handled imperfectly in health systems. But this is surely the point – it is an example of an unwinnable dilemma of public policy that gives rise to complex moral dilemmas. But to face them explicitly in the manner advocated by the rational rationers may just be too difficult and painful for society to contemplate. It denies the essentially political and value-based nature of the debate and ignores the difficulty of agreeing at a societal level a set of values that may usefully guide decision making as distinct from a set of rather banal precepts with which few would disagree but which fall woefully short as useful guides to complex decision making. The quest for rational rationing will not go away: like the other policy cleavages considered in this book, it will reappear from time to time in cyclical fashion. But this will not make it any less futile, since it is predicated on a model of social functioning that is at odds with the real world of health policy. As Mechanic succinctly puts it, 'interest in making rationing explicit arises from the illusion that optimisation is possible' (Mechanic 1995: 1659). The need is, to borrow Simon's (1957) term, to 'satisfice' in preference to seeking to optimise. The distinction is all important and offers a way through the thicket of trying to ration health care through explicit means. If in adopting such means the intention is to end the messy business of rationing health care and setting priorities, it is doomed to fail for the reasons considered in this chapter. For economists to suggest otherwise is not only naïve but betrays a lack of understanding of how complex systems work. The more likely outcome is that rationing will remain a messy affair and that at best policy makers, managers and clinicians will only be able to ameliorate its most negative features and be better placed to defend their decision making perhaps through a system of procedural rights governing the way individuals are treated and informed about decisions affecting them.

Because there is probably no realistic alternative to satisficing, whether from a practical, political or moral standpoint, concepts like accountability for reasonableness and muddling through elegantly hold appeal. This may be because they are grounded in pragmatic sensibility that has much to commend it.

SIX

Choice and competition in health systems

Introduction

Over the past two decades, choice and competition have become central planks of health policy in many countries. Such notions are in keeping with the consumerist ethos and increasing commodification of health care now prevalent in health system reform thinking and noted in earlier chapters. Of course, it is quite possible to have choice without competition, and competition without allowing choice. However, the two are generally regarded as going hand in hand, since choice without competition may result in people not having a sufficient range of options from which to choose – the problem of choosing any colour as long as it is black. Competition without choice is seen as unworkable unless there is a mechanism whereby people not only exercise voice if they do not perceive themselves to be getting a good service, but can also exit by taking their health problems elsewhere. For these reasons, these two central planks of health reform have been coupled for the purposes of this chapter.

Opponents of choice are invariably also opposed to competition and believe that both pose serious risks for the ethos and values of a public health service such as the NHS in the UK and threaten to destabilise the principle of universal access to care. Of course, as is discussed below, it is possible to confine competition to the public sector so that a genuinely internal market is created as distinct from a provider market that is open to both public and private providers. Indeed, Julian Le Grand, an influential health adviser to the former British Prime Minister, Tony Blair, argues that it is perfectly possible to have competition between publicly owned entities without any participation from the private sector. 'It is the presence of competition that matters, not the ownership structure of providers' (Le Grand 2007: 42). But such public as opposed to private markets appear confined to the Nordic countries and the notion has not been advocated or pursued in the UK where a health care market is being opened up to for-profit providers, including United Health, Virgin Care, Capita and Serco, and consultancies including McKinsey's, PricewaterhouseCoopers, and Ernst & Young.

Issues of choice and competition have traditionally divided those on the left and right of politics respectively. While those on the right have been advocates of both, believing that they will promote efficiency, those on the left have opposed choice and competition on the grounds that they will have a negative impact on equity. But, as Cooper and Le Grand (2007) point out, the left–right battle over choice and competition has ended with left-leaning policy makers coming round to the view that they might not be 'such a disaster'. Choice and competition have now come to be regarded by many on the left as having a 'potential positive impact … on equity'. They have been persuaded by advisers such as Le Grand that choice and competition offer 'better quality and less inequity than traditionally collectivist public health systems' (Cooper and Le Grand 2007: 18). Many on the left are puzzled by their colleagues' sudden conversion. They still believe that choice is associated with individualism and autonomy while equity is associated with collectivism and social justice. Regarding one as dependent on the other is akin to mixing oil and water.

So what do choice and competition actually mean and entail in a publicly funded system of health care such as the British NHS? Are they real or a deceit? Do they, as their progenitors believe, empower those who have traditionally not had choice in health services or the benefits of competition in offering that choice? Or rather do they reinforce and deepen inequalities already evident in health systems, which those same policy makers say they want to confront and arrest if not eliminate? Such questions are hotly contested, much in the manner suggested by Alford's framework described in Chapter One. Turning to the evidence base – such as it is – for answers does not help much.

Once again, the strength of belief both for and against choice and competition owes more to ideology, values and political beliefs than to the science or evidence base, which at best remains equivocal and can be used in support of almost any position. This remains the case following the coalition government's massive NHS upheaval in 2010, which was predicated on the view that more choice and competition would serve as liberating forces and improve efficiency and quality. The evidence base to support the changes is weak at best.

This chapter reviews the arguments on both sides and concludes that in systems such as the NHS choice and competition may amount to something of a deceit and a distraction. This is especially so if the view taken is that markets and medicine do not mix well. Moreover, as a result of the considerable influence of advisers and consultants, as discussed in Chapters One and Four, choice and competition are advanced as the only alternatives to dealing with underperforming and inefficient health systems. In Chapter Seven, and on the basis of the critique offered below, this argument is challenged and an alternative approach is proposed.

The appeal of markets

As the account of health system reform offered in Chapter Four shows, governments in a number of countries have resorted to market mechanisms in the belief that they will secure improved efficiency and higher quality of care through allowing choice for users and competition to drive up standards. That, after all, is what international bodies like the World Bank and Internal Monetary Fund (IMF), and the major management consultancies that advise governments, insist is required to ensure success and get results. It is the neoliberal business model applied to public services. A stark illustration of this model being ruthlessly applied has been the austerity measures imposed on Greece by the European Union, European Central Bank and IMF (the Troika) over the past five years or so with more of the same called for despite their complete failure to rescue the economy using market mechanisms to improve public services (Sen 2015).

In the Netherlands, reforms to the health care system over the past decade have been summed up as 'more market and less – but better – government' (Kraanen and Meerkerk (2006). Echoing the principles of new public management (NPM) and the work of writers such as Osborne and Gaebler (1993), reform proposals have included 'a shift in decision-making power from government to the market, deregulation of planning and tariffs, greater competition between health insurers and between care providers, greater consumer influence, and the introduction of financial incentives for all stakeholders' (Kraanen and Meerkerk 2006: 5). To prevent market failure, the government remains responsible for providing certain safeguards and ensuring that the public interest is upheld. Central to the changes in the Dutch health care system is a belief in competition and incentives, since without these there would be little or no incentive to perform well or improve standards. 'Professional ethics, pride and honour', it is claimed, though much in evidence in the Dutch system, are insufficient to meet future challenges.

Since the health care system in the Netherlands has always scored well in international comparisons and since the health of the population is generally high by international standards, it seems to be a case of all things being relative. For instance, the performance of health care in the Netherlands in terms of effectiveness and patient safety is above average for a number of indicators (Westert and Verkleij 2006). Clearly, Dutch health system reformers believe they could do better still but only if they adopt the choice and competition package on offer globally. Part of the justification for change is a perception that the concept of solidarity or mutuality is declining as people become more individualised and less willing to support collective endeavours. Yet, solidarity is still regarded as an important value and principle underlying health care provision. A challenge for the government lies in how far it can reconcile complicated issues involving the introduction of effective, but regulated, market competition while at the same time maintaining solidarity. In addition, the particular weaknesses of the Dutch system, which are by no means exclusive to it, are seen to lie in the areas of patient safety, integrated care pathways and the effectiveness of prevention and care.

Given some of the issues considered in the previous chapter, it is not immediately obvious how choice and competition can contribute to significant improvement in these areas.

Le Grand believes there are three principal arguments in favour of choice and competition as a model for public service delivery in areas such as health and education. 'It fulfils the principle of autonomy, and promotes responsiveness to users' needs and wants; it provides incentives for providers to provide both higher quality and greater efficiency; and it is likely to be more equitable than the alternatives' (Le Grand 2007: 42). In the context of centre-left governments, analysts and advisers, choice is sold on the grounds that it provides a way of addressing the problem of inequity in public services that, albeit committed to equity, end up becoming distorted by the tendency of such services to favour the articulate and confident – as Le Grand puts it, 'privileging the better off' (2007: 44). Indeed, New Labour's embrace of choice and competition is based on the concepts' potential to promote equity and improved services for users in lower socioeconomic groups. According to these newfound enthusiasts for choice and competition, the flaw in the argument of those on the old left who subscribe to collectivist public services on the grounds that they are inherently equitable is that, whatever the theory may say, in practice the services are not equitable. Certain privileged groups can in effect ensure that they exercise choice even in a system allegedly available to all without formal choice mechanisms. It is tackling such systemic bias that leads analysts/advisers such as Le Grand and Stevens to claim that the equity implications of choice-based reforms hold out more promise than the collectivist structure they are replacing.

Yet, as has been pointed out, the case for choice increasing equity has principally been made by the former and current prime ministers, a few health ministers and their advisers, a handful of recent policy statements and by a few academics (Barr et al 2008; Pollock et al 2011). But the problem with the shift to choice as a means of tackling inequity is that it makes many assumptions about both the causes of inequity and the optimal policy response to tackling them. Critics of the argument that choice leads to improved equity claim that encouraging explicit choice 'might further empower those with greater voice' (Barr et al 2008: 273). Indeed, the only evidence ever cited by the choice advocates is the London Patient Choice Pilot, which showed that the uptake of choice was the same across primary care trusts of varying levels of deprivation. But such a conclusion is not supported by other evidence, notably the scoping review commissioned by the NIHR Service Delivery and Organisation R&D programme (now known as the Health Services and Delivery Research programme) (Fotaki et al 2005). Indeed, Fotaki and her colleagues commenting on the London Patient Choice Pilot evaluation note that several disadvantaged groups were excluded from participation in the study, suggesting that its findings should be viewed accordingly and treated with caution. A second review by the Social Market Foundation similarly concluded that there was a lack of definitive evidence to indicate the extent to which socioeconomic factors influence the take-up of choice (Williams and Rossiter 2004). Having reviewed all the evidence from several countries, Fotaki and colleagues concluded that 'the impact of choice on equity is consistently negative ... Providing more choice increases inequity. This is partly because the better off are more able to exercise choice when it is offered.... At the very least, choice policies have the potential to increase inequity' (2005: 117-8). The response from the pro-choice commentators is to allay such fears by proposing patient advocacy schemes or advisers to assist patients who are from deprived groups and unfamiliar with exercising choice with making the best choice for them. But another constraint on choice is the issue of capacity; in a publicly funded system this will always be an issue as excess capacity is discouraged. Choice demands spare capacity.

Despite the absence of convincing evidence concerning the exercise of choice to improve people's health, there has been no let-up in the pursuit of the choice agenda. The coalition government's health reforms put increased choice and control at their heart. 'People want choice', the 2010 White Paper proclaimed starkly (Secretary of State for Health 2010b: paragraph 2.17: 16), without offering any insights into what is meant by choice and how other aspects of healthcare provision may count for more in a given situation. The government was critical of its Labour predecessor for having made insufficient progress on introducing patient choice and wanted to go much further in extending it to include any qualified (changed from 'willing' in the White Paper) provider. Indeed, the Health and Social Care Act 2012 requires clinical commissioning groups (CCGs) to put services out to competitive tender under the controversial section 75. It is this section above all that has led critics to claim that the NHS is on an irreversible path towards privatisation (Hunter 2013). Indeed, Lord Owen, who was a health minister in the Labour government in the mid-1970s, has predicted that 'the end of the NHS as we have known and understood it in England will take place before 2020 if whichever party or parties that win the 2015 general election does not change the 2012 NHS legislation' (Owen 2014: 260). Given that the Conservative Party won a narrow victory in the election, it seems that Owen's worst fears may be realised.

Building on the previous government's programme of personal health budget pilots, the coalition government sought to encourage further pilots and also to introduce a right to a personal health budget in discrete areas such as NHS continuing care. In *The National Health Service Five Year Forward View*, there is a commitment to making good on the NHS's promise to give patients choice over where and how they receive care (NHS England 2014). There is also a proposal to introduce integrated personal commissioning (IPC), 'a new voluntary approach to blending health and social care funding for individuals with complex needs' (NHS England 2014: 13). IPC will provide an integrated 'year of care' budget that will be managed by individuals themselves or on their behalf by local councils, the NHS or a voluntary organisation.

Patient choice, like competition, is promoted as a means for achieving greater efficiency and improved quality as well as being something that patients intrinsically value. But how far these assumptions are valid in the context of how choice works in practice and what types of choice matter to patients merits further exploration. In her critique of market-based patient choice, Fotaki identifies four key issues that need to be considered: the evidence that patient choice improves efficiency and quality is limited at best while also having negative consequences for equity, as noted above; people might be interested in different choices from those favoured by policy makers and these may be rooted in a preference for shared decision making between patient and professional rather than displaying behaviour typical of consumers in a marketplace; although choice over when, where and how care is provided might be valued, patients may be willing to trade these off against good quality services that are locally provided; and choice needs to occur in a context of support being available on the part of a trusted professional who is able to guide and advise as necessary (Fotaki 2014). Fotaki concludes on the basis of her review that the assumptions underpinning policy have been found wanting and that their applicability to health care is either limited or invalid. An unlikely ally can be found in the Secretary of State for Health, Jeremy Hunt. He has expressed the view that patient choice is not the main driver of performance improvement given that health provision often includes natural monopolies (West 2014).

A variant of choice is personalisation and it may be that what those seeking health care are really after, and want, is the latter. One of the leading architects of personalisation, Charles Leadbeater, believes that while users of public services want to be treated well, it does not mean that they want to behave like consumers shopping around for the best deal (Leadbeater 2004). It is clear from this description of personalisation that the choices Leadbeater supports are different in kind from those implied by a traditional consumer model. In particular, he is not concerned with competition. However, in 2008 the prime minister, Gordon Brown, seemed less inclined to regard such distinctions as valid. In a major speech on the future of the NHS, he asserted that 'the NHS of the future will be more than a universal service – it will be a personal service too' (Brown 2008). To emphasise the point, elsewhere in the same speech, he stated that the NHS is 'here for all of us but personal to each of us'. But it is clear from his speech that he sees competition and choice as being essential accompaniments to personalisation.

It would seem, therefore, that while an important distinction can be made between choice and personalisation, they are sometimes confused and conflated notions. It is possible to have personalisation without choice, although some of the advocates of choice consider that the push for personalisation can only come from an element of competition and choice. But pure notions of professionalism and the public service ethic place a lot of emphasis on providing services that meet the specific individual needs of users in ways that respect their dignity and their differences and varied circumstances. It would, conversely, also be possible to exercise choice in a context where the options available did not pay heed to the notion of personalisation.

A belief in, and embrace of, markets and competition has deeper roots. There is, in particular, Bobbitt's assertion, cited in Chapter One, that market states are replacing welfare states in an age of globalisation where nation states are fighting for their survival and retention of their identity. Whether such replacement is inevitable or unavoidable remains to be seen but the past decade or so has witnessed a reawakening of nationalism in many countries as evidenced by support for the Scottish National Party in Scotland, and the rise of left-wing parties in Greece and Spain opposed to austerity and to the privatisation of the public realm. Then there is the growing influence of neoliberalism, which gained a foothold in the UK and elsewhere in the 1970s and is seemingly impervious to changes of government (Gray 2007). During this period, the welfare state came under attack, aided by the confluence of a variety of economic, demographic and ideological factors. Paradoxically, the welfare state was no longer regarded as the solution for economic problems but as one of its causes (Timmins 1995). The appeal of markets grew as they were deemed the most appropriate agents to ensure the provision of efficient services that best met individuals' needs. During the 1990s, 'the golden era of expansion turned into the era of accountability, control and attempted retrenchment' (Marmor et al 1990: 29). Anti-welfare ideas originated in the US, spread to the UK and to other countries in Europe and beyond. As Ranade (1998), Gauld (2001) and Maarse (2004) among others described the spread of such ideas, several countries including New Zealand, Australia, the Netherlands, Sweden, and Germany joined the search for ways to reduce the role of government in health care and increase the role of the private sector in the belief that it performed better. In New Zealand, for example, during the late 1980s and 1990s, the combined theories of public choice, new institutional economics and new public management provided a 'potent cocktail' for policy makers. As Gauld describes the then fourth Labour government's public sector reform strategy, 'the overriding assumption which policy makers extracted from [these] theories is that markets are the "natural" place in which services – public or private – should be delivered' (2001: 43). It was a belief driven by a conviction that markets, together with the competition and incentives they facilitate, are more efficient and innovative than other models. Market creation could entail corporatising, privatising or contracting out of services. Such mechanisms have characterised health systems in many countries since this period.

Neoliberals believe in limited government and strong unfettered markets – the coalition government's policy thrust on various fronts was arguably deliberately designed to shrink the state. As two analysts argued shortly after the coalition government took office, 'the coalition programme ... involves a restructuring of ... public services that takes the country in a new direction, rolling back the state to a level of intervention below that in the United States – something which is unprecedented. Britain will abandon the goal of attaining a European level of public provision. The policies include substantial privatisation and a shift of responsibility from state to individual' (Taylor-Gooby and Stoker 2011: 14). The Conservative government elected in May 2015 is determined to maintain that course, which should come as no surprise since it is prominent Conservatives, notably Oliver Letwin and John Redwood, who, alongside Andrew Lansley, were behind the NHS reforms of 2010. They have long regarded the NHS's flaws and deficiencies as ones that could only be tackled through opening the service up to competition and market forces (Letwin and Redwood 1988). No evidence to the contrary has dimmed their view of what needs to be done. Had it done so, the Health and Social Care Act 2012 would have been a very different piece of legislation or might not have existed at all.

Such staunch neoliberal believers regard the advance of the free market as an unstoppable historical process. Paradoxically, however, the construction of such markets in housing, education, health and other sectors has required strong and highly centralised government to coerce people and institutions into accepting and implementing the reforms desired by ministers. It seems strangely ironic if we are denied a choice about choice because it is deemed good for us! Freeing up the market, far from diminishing the role of the state or shrinking its size, has actually led to a strengthening of central government power. Permeating neoliberal thinking is a belief in what the late Hugo Young called 'the business imperative as the sole agent of economic recovery' (quoted in Gray 2007: 79). Such a business imperative was also believed to be the salvation of underperforming public services, as is evident from the reports emanating from businessmen brought in by government over the years to advise on public service reform. In the NHS, the influence of Roy Griffiths in the 1980s and Derek Wanless in the early years of the 21st century spring to mind.

Although Margaret Thatcher's embrace of neoliberalism when she was prime minister of a Conservative government during the 1980s and early 1990s was perhaps not so surprising in the Britain she sought to create in the 1980s, New Labour's embrace of it was less obvious at the time, although, with hindsight, it seemed a logical move. As Gray puts it, 'once in power it was clear Blair came not to bury Thatcher but to continue her work' (2007: 94). He 'swallowed Thatcher's faith in the market as an elixir that would revivify the party and bring it back to power' (Gray 2007: 85). Blair, together with his chancellor (later prime minister), Gordon Brown, accepted neoliberal economics and the two men were the chief architects of New Labour and all it stood for.

As a consequence, neoliberal ideas shaped policy in Britain, and many other countries in the late 1980s, and continue to do so (Paton 2014). The concept of NPM, described at some length in Chapter Two, has been a manifestation of this way of thinking in respect of public service reform. During the Blair years, neoliberalism became entwined with the modernisation mantra that meant 'the reorganisation of society around the imperatives of the free market' (Gray 2007: 94).

Critics who took issue with this belief inevitably became branded as regressive and stuck in the past. They were seen as hankering after a bygone golden age of collectivism and solidarity that was now regarded as responsible for inferior and insensitive public services that no longer met the requirements of a generation that had become used to other 'isms', notably individualism and consumerism. After a faltering start when his government appeared to be rolling back the preceding Conservative government's public service changes, Blair carried on the agenda of privatisation started by Thatcher and went much further in respect of introducing market mechanisms into the NHS. The journey began in the late 1980s with the arrival of the internal market in the NHS, which had its parallels in many other countries as diverse as the Netherlands, Sweden and New Zealand. It pursued its logical path during the late 1990s and into the first decade of the 21st century. The change of government in 1997 gave rise to a brief pause on the journey, but not to a change of direction that successive governments have pursued with determination and mounting vigour ever since.

The limits to markets

The limits to markets in health care are well documented, especially in the classic article by the economist Kenneth Arrow (Arrow 1963), but also by more recent respected authorities like Michael Sandel, who argues that a 'debate about the moral limits of markets would enable us to decide, as a society, where markets serve the public good and where they don't belong' (Sandel 2013: 14). The limits to markets were usefully and persuasively summarised in a lecture Gordon Brown gave to the Social Market Foundation (SMF) in 2003 when he was Chancellor of the Exchequer (Brown 2004). In the manner of his predecessor as prime minister, Tony Blair, Brown made the reform of the NHS one of his major priorities, and so his views on markets and medicine might have seemed significant and suggested that he would seek to move the NHS reform programme in a different direction. In practice, there were few signs of such a shift occurring up until Labour lost the election in 2010. In his 2003 speech, Brown referred to the asymmetry of information between the producer and the consumer as patient, which meant that the consumer was unable to seek out the best product at the lowest price or to access complete information – as is possible in a conventional market. As a result, the risk of market failure could be serious. Brown went on to describe the features of the NHS – or, indeed, any health system – that would make it difficult to commercialise, namely:

- the need for guaranteed security of supply, which means that a local hospital could not be allowed to go out of business;
- the need also for clusters of mutually reinforcing specialties;
- a high volume of work to guarantee quality of service;
- the economies of scale and scope making it difficult to tackle these market failures by market solutions;
- the difficulty for private sector contracts in anticipating and specifying the range of essential characteristics that users demand of a health care system.

Summarising why health is different from other sectors, Brown listed the following:

- price signals do not always work;
- the consumer is not always sovereign;
- there is potential abuse of monopoly power;
- it is hard to write and enforce contracts;
- it is difficult to let a hospital go bust;
- there is a risk of supplier induced demand.

Brown conceded that the private sector had a limited role in routine procedures in health care and in promoting contestability. He also maintained it had a role 'where private capacity does not simply replace NHS capacity' (Brown 2004: 27). He saw no role for the private sector in those areas where 'complex medical conditions and uncertain needs make it virtually impossible to capture them in the small print of contracts' (Brown 2004: 27).

Brown concluded his analysis of market failure by proposing that the reform and modernisation of the public realm did not need to rely on market mechanisms but should be achieved through devolution, transparency and accountability. He maintained that 'the assumption that the only alternative to command and control is a market means of public service delivery has obscured the real challenge in health care' (Brown 2004: 30). He went on: 'it is only by developing decentralised non market models for public provision ... that we will show to those who assert that whatever the market failure the state failure will always be greater, that a publicly funded and provided service can deliver efficiency, equity and be responsive to the consumer' (Brown 2004: 30).

Coming from one of the principal architects of the public service modernisation project, perhaps it is not so odd that despite such a clear-eyed analysis of the limits to markets in health policy and a powerful endorsement of a public service model, the government in England under Brown's premiership not only continued to give credence to market-style solutions but also offered positive encouragement to the commercial sector and its expansion into the NHS. Indeed, in a blatant disregard of the position he adopted in his 2003 SMF speech, Brown firmly endorsed the direction of travel set out by Blair and successive health ministers in his first major speech on the NHS since taking over as prime minister, delivered in January 2008. The speech is peppered with references to the importance of competition, choice and diversity of supply in improving health and health care (Brown 2008). He made it clear that reform should go further and that individual budgets for patients should be introduced and, after successful piloting, rolled out nationally – as noted earlier, a policy readily embraced by the coalition government in 2010. Initially, such budgets would be an extension of those already operating in social care and would be available to people with long-term conditions. However, one of the principal proponents of such budgets – Julian Le Grand once again – believes that direct payments in health care could be extended to other areas such as maternity services (Le Grand 2007).

Direct payments are claimed to bring various benefits, including incentives for improving provider performance and empowering patients through increasing their range of choice of provider and/ or treatment. Most important is the belief that patient budgets can improve patients' health and well-being. But it is not a case of all gain and no pain. For example, one critic of patient budgets, who is also a service user activist, is worried that major issues of principle have yet to be properly acknowledged, let alone thought through (Beresford 2008). First, Beresford sees little difference between the health vouchers advocated by Thatcher's neoliberal ideologues in the 1980s and early 1990s and individual budgets being promoted by Labour ministers and by the then prime minister, Gordon Brown. Beresford wonders if individual budgets might weaken the NHS and the universal principle on which it is predicated. How is the circle to be squared between a service still largely free at the point of use and a model of cash payments? Moreover, what will be included as part of people's individual health budget, and what will continue to be part of their core NHS entitlement? What will stop the latter being eaten away? And what will happen to individual budgets if governments or economic circumstances get harsher? None of these questions has gone away or been satisfactorily answered despite the efforts of more recent governments and NHS England to extend such policies.

The rhetoric of markets and the engagement of the private sector in stimulating them in the NHS was given added impetus with the passage of the Health and Social Care Act 2012, the impact of which is still being felt in the NHS. The Act marked the final step in the creation of an external market for NHS care and one underpinned by numerous contracts held between the NHS and the private providers of healthcare. It has been estimated that the NHS contracts out the provision of services to the private sector to the tune of over £20 billion a year, or a fifth of the total healthcare budget, with the 'newest and biggest area of outsourcing' occurring in those services that the NHS used to provide directly, namely, community health services and secondary care (Centre for Health and the Public Interest 2015). The case for outsourcing made by ministers and other politicians is that it provides a route to better and cheaper public services. But the evidence to support such assertions is woefully lacking (Coote and Penny 2014).

Indeed, the review conducted by the Centre for Health and the Public Interest concluded that the NHS is 'poorly equipped to ensure that healthcare services outsourced to for-profit providers will provide safe, high-quality care and good value for money' (Centre for Health and the Public Interest 2015, paragraph 8: 5). In their painstaking study stretching back over 30 years to the arrival of new public management, Hood and Dixon found that as a consequence of outsourcing public services, 'far from falling, running costs rose substantially in absolute terms over thirty years, while complaints soared' (Hood and Dixon 2015: 178).

Such a conclusion is strikingly at odds with the political rhetoric claiming that outsourcing improves the performance of public services at lower cost. What may be a more accurate description of what has been happening is provided by Wilks, who has highlighted the 'colonisation' of the UK state by powerful private corporations both as entrenched for-profit providers of large and increasing swathes of public services, including the NHS, and as a key part of the governance of departments and agencies, supplying board members and senior personnel (Wilks 2013). Furthermore, such private sector bodies have been skilled lobbyists, advancing their interests and doing so by, among other things, financing political parties' electoral campaigns. The result is public policy formation that reflects the interests and preferences of such bodies rather than those of the voters and taxpayers (Jones 2015). The phenomenon has been termed 'institutional corruption' (Draca 2014), but also fits Pollitt's portrayal of managerialism in public services as an ideology rather than a pragmatic response, whereby true believers need no evidence-based results to prove the correctness of their ideas (Pollitt 1993). Rather, it is a case of hope triumphing over evidence.

Should we be concerned about what some perceive to be a 'hollowing out' of public services? Perhaps not, if they were functioning better and at lower cost than those they replaced. But since it seems they are not, should there be closer public scrutiny of what might seem to be a form of insidious corruption alive and well within the British state? There are those, including the King's Fund and its chief economist, John Appleby, and other think tanks on both the centre left and right, that believe that ownership of the means of production is not really the issue – what matters is the quality of care and management and these would apply regardless of whether the service was publically or privately delivered.

While this is all true, is it as simple as that, given what we know about the lack of evidence in regard to outsourcing and the neoliberal political ideology that seems to be driving policy? Perhaps ownership does matter, especially when ensuring that effective contracting and regulatory processes are in place seems so problematic. Commissioning has remained largely undeveloped and has failed to live up to the hopes and expectations of its advocates (Hunter and Williams 2012; Smith et al 2013). Indeed, with moves towards integrated care being actively encouraged, we may be witnessing the demise of commissioning which has existed in one form or another since 1990 but which is increasingly at odds with the purchaser–provider split (Jupp 2015).

Returning to Alford's framework, introduced in Chapter One as a way of aiding an understanding of health policy, it is possible to view the events that have occurred in recent decades through the lens of his notion of structural interests and his opposing groups of reformers – those labelled 'market reformers' on the one hand, and 'bureaucratic reformers' on the other. Since the 1980s, market reformers have clearly been in the ascendant; of the three groups of structural interests, it is the challenging corporate and managerial interests that have been dominant. The dominant professional interest and the repressed community interest, while uneasy about the direction taken by the reforms, have remained remarkably pliant. However, the lack of public reaction by these interests should not be construed as an indication of quiet acceptance, even if many are gloomily resigned to what they regard as inevitable and feel powerless to prevent it. The reforms have left deep scars. As Harrison concludes from his three-country study of implementing health changes, 'market reform helped undermine established forms of discourse, thinking, and practice among health managers and professionals' (2004: 187). In particular, the administrative and professional mindsets that had dominated health care policy and practice from the 1960s through to the early 1980s 'began to give way to more business and market-oriented discourse and thinking' (Harrison 2004: 187).

Of Harrison's three countries, the UK was the most ambitious in its attempt to introduce such changes. The approach in the Netherlands and Sweden was more gradual, in part because neither country had such a centralised, command and control system of government that allowed it to act in such a decisive, unilateral manner. As Harrison notes, the market-style changes were felt most sharply among managers and least dramatically among professionals. He maintains that the market reforms 'had very little impact on many important features of subcultures of hospital and ambulatory physicians' (Harrison 2004: 187). Moreover, 'professional norms, assumptions, and practices remained largely unchanged in crucial fields like specialty training, clinical practice, peer supervision, professional ethics, research and relations among specialties' (Harrison 2004: 187). It was also the case that many clinicians decided to focus on their clinical work and distance themselves from senior management and the priorities being determined by government. In so doing, they became increasingly cynical of and embittered by managers and policy makers. This, in turn, made it difficult for the government to proceed to implement its ambitious changes in the future direction of health care.

In particular, the government wanted to see more health care offered by primary and community care services as an alternative to expensive inpatient hospital care. It also wanted to give a higher priority to health prevention and to narrowing the health gap between rich and poor. However, in the pursuit of such worthy goals, it was by no means self-evident that the successive waves of structural and organisational reforms that swept over the NHS from the 1980s would have a material impact on such matters. Indeed, it may be that they have principally served as a major and unhelpful distraction from addressing such concerns. This is certainly the conclusion of a review of the government's record over the past decade in tackling health inequalities (Dowler and Spencer 2007a). Notwithstanding some important achievements, like the reductions in child poverty and the introduction of the minimum wage and its uprating, 'key fundamental drivers such as income distribution have worsened over the decade' (Dowler and Spencer 2007b: 235). The position has deteriorated further since then, especially in the North of England (Whitehead 2014).

In terms of who has benefited most from the market reforms, both in the UK and elsewhere, it seems clear at first sight that managers probably gained most, both materially and in terms of additional power (or perhaps more accurately, perceived or symbolic power, since the real power has remained with the government throughout). However, on closer inspection, it may be that managers have deluded themselves that they have been the chief beneficiaries of the government's reforms. The Faustian bargain struck was that managers' elevated position came at a heavy price – progressively they became conduits for doing the government's bidding and in fact enjoyed reduced autonomy and flexibility to determine the destiny of the organisation and services they oversaw (Blackler 2006).

Reporting on his interviews with NHS chief executives, Blackler concludes that 'while there was more rhetoric than ever about the importance of leadership, in practice, chief executives were being given less space to lead' (2006: 12). Contributing factors were 'too many central prescriptions, unrealistic expectations for "quick wins" and the development of a culture of bullying' (2006: 12). Paradoxically, despite its apparent enthusiasm for management, the government was 'deeply mistrustful of chief executives and [was] unfairly scapegoating them for the shortcomings of the system' (Blackler 2006: 13). Claims to be working 'in a climate of fear' were not uncommon. Such findings led Blackler to conclude that 'the popular image of empowered, proactive leaders has little relevance to the work of the NHS chief executive in the UK' (2006: 19). The government's approach to running the NHS had more in common with Taylorism than with contemporary approaches to management – approaches that the government insisted it wanted to introduce and support. However, as was shown in Chapter Four, such developments were at odds with the introduction of market-style thinking into the NHS, since it might be assumed that such an approach would encourage the emergence of entrepreneurial managers who would be accorded the space and freedom to innovate and develop services in new ways to meet the government's objectives of providing more efficient and responsive services. But the severe financial pressures on the NHS appear to have put paid to that freedom. The future of foundation trusts is in doubt and chief executives are leaving the NHS in worrying numbers as their hospitals are put into special measures following the failure to balance the books.

Perhaps the most surprising aspect of the ongoing debate over markets and medicine is the absence of convincing or unequivocal evidence at a time when government was firmly wedded to an evidence-based approach to policy. The mantra when it entered office in 1997 was that it did not matter who provided services or who did what as long as it worked. But, as in other areas of public policy, the evidence is equivocal and contested. Each side of the argument can carefully select and cite evidence in support of its particular thesis. As we have noted, advocates of choice and competition, such as Le Grand (2007), Porter and Teisberg (2006) and Smith (2006), cite evidence to demonstrate that carefully managed and regulated competition in which proper attention is paid to incentives can increase improvements in care. Moreover, they believe that encouraging competition from the independent sector can be a spur to improved efficiency in existing NHS provision. The problem is establishing cause and effect and attributing precise changes to the impact of competition rather than to some other influence or development that may in fact have little directly to do with the health care system but with the quality of housing, the state of the labour market or some other contributor to improved health. Moreover, it is one thing to subscribe to an economics textbook view of markets and how they operate and quite another to examine the dynamics of competition and markets in the real, messy world of politics. And in health systems, the politics do not come much messier – a point returned to later.

Of course, the proponents of choice and competition remain convinced that their arguments are sound and right. Porter and Teisberg (2006) take as their starting point the failure of competition in the US health care system, as evident in the provision of services that are high in cost, low in quality and do not benefit patients. Their thesis is not that competition may be bad and that an NHS-type system is therefore needed (though many in the US do believe that precisely such a cure is needed), but that 'value based competition on results at the right level' is what is needed. Justifying their stance, they write:

> It simply strains credibility to imagine that a large government entity would streamline administration, simplify prices, set prices according to true costs, help patients make choices based on excellence and value, establish value based competition at the provider level and make politically neutral and tough choices to deny patients and reimbursement to sub-standard providers ... (Porter and Teisberg 2006: 89)

Yet, in many ways this is precisely what the government in England is seeking to do in respect of its reforms. Moreover, even if a different system were introduced of the type Porter and Teisberg propose, it is inconceivable that the political issues referred to would not arise. It is extremely naive to assume that government can, and will, withdraw from health care provision. Indeed, the evidence is all to the contrary, with governments becoming more involved in health care rather than less. But Porter and Teisberg favour a transformation of health care in such a way that it realigns competition with value for patients. 'Value in health care is the health outcome per dollar of cost expended. If all system participants have to compete on value, value will improve dramatically. As simple and obvious as this seems to be, however, improving value has not been the central goal of participants in the system' (Porter and Teisberg 2006: 4).

Smith believes that the chances of bringing about such a competitive system are higher in the UK than in the US, since he somewhat glibly dismisses the 'opponents of change' as being 'the ideologues of the left and the public sector unions – but their power will weaken in the face of patients demanding choice on the back of good and available information' (Smith 2006: 26). He believes that opposition in the US will be harder to overcome because of the power of the vested commercial interests. For Smith, the answer to public sector involvement is not private sector involvement per se. Rather, it is the need to challenge the monopolistic abuse of power through the introduction of competition. It would be possible, for instance, to have a genuine internal provider market within the public sector, as in Sweden. Although Smith does not explicitly mention such an option, it would be one that would satisfy his belief that a dysfunctional system is unlikely to be radically changed by those within in who have profited from it and built their careers by being successful within it. Le Grand, however, as mentioned near the start of the chapter, does acknowledge the distinction, claiming that critics of choice and competition often confuse these with the privatisation of services. It is, as he argues, quite possible to have competition between publicly owned or non-profit entities without any participation from the private sector, since it is the presence of competition that matters and not the ownership of providers.

Yet, as was also noted earlier, it does appear to be the case that when choice and competition are invoked as desirable policy instruments, it is the for-profit private sector that is usually envisaged as the means whereby such a market will be created. The Swedish model of the planned market is not one that has greatly influenced reform in other countries. Certainly, in the English NHS, which may be regarded as a hybrid version of a planned market, apart from the occasional mention of not-for-profit social enterprises, the new entrants to the health care market are from the commercial sector and have headquarters that are usually overseas. A planned market:

> involves the intentional creation of a new market through the exercise of state power. This market can be consciously designed to achieve state policy objectives through limited and selected use of market instruments. Planned (unlike regulated) markets typically include a substantial number of publicly owned and operated competitors, increasing the leverage of public policy-makers while limiting the impact of the private capital market. (Saltman and von Otter 1992: 17)

Only Northern Europe has attempted to generate competitive conditions inside a wholly publicly capitalised delivery system – what Saltman and von Otter term 'public competition'. The model being developed in the UK's NHS comes closer to what Saltman and von Otter call 'a neo-classically influenced mixed market' (1992: 37). The reasons for Britain taking a different direction in respect of its public sector reform journey lie, Saltman and von Otter believe, in Britain's political culture being much more individualistic despite the existence of the welfare state and the NHS and therefore more responsive to market types of thinking than is the case in respect of Nordic countries with their more collectivist philosophical roots. Public competition is designed to offer the benefits of market-style systems of health care, such as patient voice and choice, with none of its disadvantages, such as cost inflation, cream skimming or rising inequalities.

The difficulty with Smith's thesis, and that of those who hold similar views and argue in similar terms, is that its unswerving faith in the for-profit marketplace and in unrestrained competition that will allow the invisible hand to work to enable patients to exercise choice in their best interests fails completely to acknowledge where health care may be different from other sectors and where the logic of the market may not apply. It may be fashionable to view patients as consumers, but ill people (who consume most care) are unlikely to be able to shop around no matter how good or accessible the information available. Nor are they well placed to appraise quality – they look for support, guidance and advice from professionals. In Smith's ideal world of health care, none of these inconvenient truths seems to be present. Indeed, they are not even acknowledged but are simply airbrushed out of the model he presents. But this is the real, messy world in which health care is provided and where neat models that work on paper rarely make the transition unscathed and are little more than caricatures. Either that, or they are aimed at the 'worried well', whose need, as distinct from demand, for health care is limited.

Advocates of the market also fail even to acknowledge, let alone address, the evidence that markets lead to sharp increases in administrative costs, as has occurred in the UK and New Zealand since the introduction of market mechanisms. As Woolhandler and Himmelstein (2007: 1127) put it, 'the decision to unleash market forces is, among other things, a decision to divert healthcare dollars to paperwork'. Another commentator, in similar vein, suggests that the introduction of markets into public sector organisations 'has merely led to an explosion in administration costs as cooperation between departments is replaced by everybody trying to invoice each other for their services' (Craig 2006: 17). Marketing services is another huge cost that may add little of value to health care or its outcomes. Yet, since April 2008, cash-strapped hospitals in England are able, within fairly general guidelines produced by the Department of Health, to market their services to increase custom and income.

The belief among many market advocates is that market forces can be put to good use, provided the incentives are properly conceived and implemented (Dixon et al 2003). Le Grand, for example, and as noted earlier, supports the introduction and development of stronger market incentives to improve performance among secondary care providers. However, fellow economist, Peter Smith (2003), disagrees with such thinking and does not support even modest experimentation with stronger market incentives, drawing attention to the adverse effects that market incentives can produce in health care. He also suggests that market disciplines could seriously undermine the professional ethic in health care, resulting in poorer quality care and health outcomes for patients.

The professional ethic could be crucial because, as Smith states, contracts can never be complete. Professional norms therefore play a critical role in smoothing out the inevitable imperfections in market contracts, and intervention to adjust them needs to be exercised with extreme care. This is an important and underexplored issue that merits further attention and research. Whereas economists tend to focus on information and incentives as the principal devices to achieve improved performance, a third determinant of behaviour, long recognised by sociologists, centres on the intrinsic objectives of personnel. As Smith and others such as Degeling and colleagues (1998) have noted, professional culture is an important determinant of improved performance. It is hard to see how a competitive market will contribute to a more effective professional culture. Indeed, it may corrode such a culture and encourage the development of competitive behaviours that are counter-productive and militate against better care and health outcomes. Under such circumstances, the costs of market reforms are likely to outweigh significantly any benefits that may accrue. For Smith, the emphasis should be on 'designing appropriate incentives into terms of employment, and nurturing a professional culture of sharing experience and seeking out continuous improvement' (2003: 31). He concludes: 'true market competition introduces a set of very raw incentives that carry serious potential for adverse outcome for many aspects of health care' (Smith 2003: 31).

Finally, Smith believes that a more competitive market between secondary care providers risks focusing managers' attention on the acute sector at the expense of the non-acute. This seems especially perverse at a time when the policy emphasis is on care out of hospital and on illness prevention. Smith claims it is difficult to envisage circumstances in which a truly competitive market can be created for many common chronic conditions with complex patient needs for which there are few, if any, clear measures of outcome and where the need is for a heavy reliance on joined-up working with other agencies, notably local authorities. Competitive markets could well work against the development of effective partnerships and result in greater fragmentation of care.

Advocates of choice and competition do concede that their chances of success – and conversely the avoidance of distortions arising from problems of information asymmetry, cherry picking and adverse selection – hinge crucially on the conditions under which they are used and on the policy instruments involved being properly designed. Le Grand, for example, in claiming that choice and competition 'can deliver greater user autonomy, higher service quality, greater efficiency, greater responsiveness and greater equity than the alternatives' (2007: 45–6), insists that the word 'can' is critical. He concedes that choice and competition face problems and that many conditions have to be met to ensure that they work as intended.

Although these are matters of execution rather than principle, and markets and competition can be challenged on both counts, they are in fact major issues and not merely technicalities that are of little consequence or are quickly mentioned in passing and then quietly glossed over. They strike at the very heart of the argument and assume that perfect policy design is something governments can successfully undertake and manage. However, if the pro-choice and competition reformers consider government to be inept when it comes to designing policy and delivering services within the confines of a public sector model that are not reliant on choice and competition, why should this same government be credited with the ability to design the perfect policy when it comes to introducing market mechanisms into health systems? Certainly, the evidence suggests otherwise.

Again, Le Grand is not impervious to such criticism. Reflecting on his time working at No 10 Downing Street as the prime minister's health adviser, he says a consequence of doing so was that 'while it did not change my mind about the general merits of the choice-and-competition model as a means of delivering public services, it did sharpen my awareness of some of the problems involved in putting it into practice' (2007: 3). Indeed, throughout his book, which is a plea for more choice and competition, Le Grand is at pains to point out that his model will only achieve its desired ends 'under the right conditions' and if the 'policy instruments' are 'properly designed'. Appropriate policy design requires three conditions to be met: competition must be real, choice must be informed, and cream skimming must be avoided. But of course, these deceptively simple requirements are extremely difficult to ensure in practice, especially by governments inexperienced in regulating the private sector, as observed by Kettl (1993) among others, and commented upon further below.

A paradox of markets is the attempt by providers to dominate them and establish a monopoly or cartel in order to remove competition. Informed choice is especially difficult in health for reasons already referred to, notably the presence of information asymmetry. And, finally, cream skimming is all too often present in market-dominated settings and not at all easy to avoid or eliminate. Indeed, as has been noted, companies employ large marketing departments whose job it is to devise selective recruitment schemes to attract healthy people (Woolhandler and Himmelstein 2007). Financial incentives are used to encourage doctors to persuade sick patients to leave the health maintenance organisation. Care is focused on the modest needs of healthy (and profitable) older people. Why it should be possible to guard against such stratagems in the UK when it has been impossible to do so in the US is never addressed. Yet the issue is a very real one when many of the same companies that practise in such a manner in the US are looking to develop lucrative markets in the UK and elsewhere in Europe. There is little acknowledgement of such issues among market advocates. It seems that all the knaves lurk in the public sector while only shining knights are to be found in the private sector (Le Grand 2003).

To meet the conditions noted above to ensure perfect policy design and a smooth-running health care market with the optimal mix of choice and competition, Kettl asserts that the government's relationships with the private sector require 'aggressive management by a strong, competent government' (1993: 6). It is a myth to claim that competition always advances efficiency, as is evident from the experience in the US (see later). But Kettl goes further and alleges that many of the problems that advocates of competition rail against 'are the *result* of government's growing reliance on the private sector and its lack of capacity to manage public-private relationships' (1993: 6, emphasis in original). When it comes to managing the problems to which competition can give rise, governments are invariably weak, a situation that arises in part from government disinvesting in its own capacity and in-house expertise at the same time as it becomes more reliant on contracted-out expertise and specialist knowledge. Successive governments' experience with outsourcing, noted earlier, illustrates the problems well. The failings of governments are the result of 'incompetent awarders of contracts on the government side', who 'have often been matched with greedy and sometime incompetent contractors on the private-sector side' (King and Crewe 2014: 417). Exactly as Kettl warned, government departments were urged by the

National Audit Office and Public Accounts Committee to be 'much tougher and more astute in their dealings' with companies (King and Crewe 2014: 418). It is a weakness that is also compounded by the very nature of public service activity where the goals pursued are complex and political in origin. This results in those goals being not only complex but also often conflicting, as was discussed in Chapter Four in respect of why the public sector is different and distinctive.

There is another difficulty with markets and medicine, as we explored to some degree in the previous section in the alleged virtues of choice. This is the unlikelihood that markets can provide the kind of health care wanted based on principles of equity and efficiency (White 2007). Indeed, writing about the relationship between markets and medical care in the US, White claims that 'for any kind of "market-oriented" reform of American health care to have significantly positive effects on cost, access, and quality, it would to include such substantial restrictions on the normal ways of doing business … that it would be barely recognisable as "market oriented" in the American context' (2007: 3). The conclusion reached by White from his extensive review of the evidence regarding the development of the US health care market from 1993 to 2005 includes the following:

- 'Market incentives and behaviours by themselves do nothing to solve basic organisational problems such as how to manage complex organisations filled with professionals who have conflicting values and interests.'
- 'Market behaviour reflected fundamentals of supply and demand of potential profit only as refracted through, so sometimes distorted by, stories that were told in the health policy and investment communities.' (White 2007: 18; White notes that the frequent inaccuracy of these stories should give pause to anyone who believes the market is somehow rational and neutral in its transactions.)

Another myth of markets is that they will offer a more tempting array of choices than could possibly be provided by other arrangements. Just as such a myth has been exposed in the deregulation of the media and the spawning of multiple channels with schedules stuffed with game shows, reality shows and suchlike, so the same applies to health care. Simply offering more choices is beside the point if the choices are deemed unattractive or are not what is needed. For Meek (2014: 185) it seems that those who run our health system do not appear to 'have a clear idea of the difference between "choice" or "marketing"'. For White and other critics of markets in health care, effective reform of health systems 'will require restraining the market, not relying on it' (White 2007: 20).

Finally, despite the many alleged benefits and virtues of competition that have been challenged in this chapter, it is by its very nature disruptive to the smooth running of health services. High transaction costs, often overlooked, are imposed on both the buyer (commissioner in UK health policy parlance) and the seller (the contractor or provider). The paradox is that despite the desire for competition to improve efficiency and raise quality, competition is actually often shunned by those charged with making the system work. For them, competition is disruptive. But once the system of providing care is in place, no one has any incentive to disrupt the system. Just as the government is accused of monopolistic behaviour, the same charge can be levelled at independent contractors.

As noted earlier, good policy design is critical if competition is to achieve its desired goals and not produce perverse incentives. But, in keeping with Sennett's remark about modern governments being compulsive consumers of policy, policy making often receives more attention than policy execution. Symbolic stands can easily be taken and receive easy media attention, whereas becoming embroiled in the detail often holds far less appeal. But because policy implementation lacks the glamour and sense of discovery associated with policy making, it receives short shrift. Of course, the situation would be little different if the government were left to itself to implement services directly. Indeed, as in the case of the UK's NHS, governments (at least in England) did provide services directly. But because of growing dissatisfaction with performance, the government looked to competition and to new entrants to the market to address the problem.

In the light of these observations, arguments favouring choice and competition seem naive in the face of the success of business and corporate interests in maximising their advantage and shareholder value, and manipulating governments to ensure that their interests are not merely protected but significantly advanced. The history of private finance initiative schemes in the UK, together with the example of the privatisation of the rail network, would seem to testify to the immense difficulties governments experience once they lose control of a service or facility.

The evidence against choice and competition is also extensive and persuasive, as the review conducted by White (2007) cited above testifies. But other recent evidence can be cited, too. For example, Woolhandler and Himmelstein (2007) conclude that 'extensive research' shows that the US for-profit health institutions 'provide inferior care at inflated prices'. They warn that the poor performance of US health care 'is directly attributable to reliance on market mechanisms and for-profit firms and should warn other nations from this path' (Woolhandler and Himmelstein 2007: 1129). In particular, their message is directed at European countries where policy makers are pushing similar arrangements that mix public funding and private management. It is a mix that, the researchers allege, accounts for the 'dismal record' arising from 'health policies that emphasise market incentives' (Woolhandler and Himmelstein 2007: 1126). In their comparison of health and old age care policies in the UK and Sweden, Fotaki and Boyd (2005) observe how societal values influence policies as well as being shaped by them. Notions of privatisation, choice and competition 'reflect normative shifts from post-war values of solidarity and equality to autonomy and individualism' (Fotaki and Boyd 2005: 241). The authors claim that such trends will continue 'despite the absence of robust evidence testifying to the validity of claims of improved efficacy of market-style mechanisms in the delivery of health and old age care' (Fotaki and Boyd 2005: 241). Gloomily, they conclude that the consequence of these policy developments is that 'inequalities are likely to widen'. Levels of trust are also likely to decline, reinforced when 'tools associated with commodity exchange are introduced into an imperfect market' (Fotaki and Boyd 2005: 241). They warn that with a loss of trust could come threats to public services, since the government will not be seen to be guarantor of health. Regardless of the intentions of government, a set of forces will have been set in train, and may prove difficult to control or direct. Critics of the coalition government's reforms enshrined in the Health and Social Care Act 2012 would agree and would argue that many of these forces are already at work to the detriment of the NHS and its founding principles.

Conclusion

The thrust of health system reform in many countries has been the adoption of market-style arrangements involving choice and competition at their centre. Those opposed to, or wary of the inflated claims made for, markets in health care are often dismissed as being opposed to change, as defending outmoded professional practices and self-interest, or as reactionaries harking back to a mythical golden age (Hunter 2006c). But this is not so – or at least not in every case when an objection is raised or counter-argument advanced. Of course health systems in every country need innovation and improvement. Indeed, most, if not all, health systems already display a considerable amount of change and innovation as technological and other advances allow things to be done, often in ways that were inconceivable until recently (for example, treatment for severe mental illness, and new forms of treatment for cancers and stroke that raise survival rates). Klein once described the NHS as 'an ant-heap seething with local initiatives: a setting for countless spontaneous experiments in the organisation and delivery of health care' (1983: 163).

Perhaps the most significant argument concerning any assessment of the pros and cons of choice competition centres on the relationship between public and private. New Labour has been at pains to blur the boundary between them but is this not being disingenuous? Choice and the promise of personalised services and care 'offer to mimic the workings of market exchange in public services, though without (so far) the direct exchange of cash or its equivalents' (Clarke et al 2008: 251). With individual budgets for health care for patients with long-term conditions being introduced in England, the health care market will come to resemble a traditional market. But the important point is that 'treating public services as though they are simply transactions misses many aspects of what makes them public' (Clarke et al 2008: 251).

This is an issue to which we return in the final chapter of this book, as it is central to what it means to finance and deliver health and health care through public means. At issue is whether it is necessary to look to markets and the for-profit sector as the only or principal means to provide such innovation and improvement. Or are policy makers being hopelessly seduced and duped, either ignoring the inconvenient evidence to the contrary or being highly selective in its application? Woolhandler and Himmelstein firmly believe it is the latter, since in their view the evidence shows unequivocally that 'remedies imported from commerce consistently yield inferior care at inflated prices' (2007: 1128). Put bluntly in their words: 'only a dunce could believe that market based reform will improve efficiency or effectiveness' (p 1128). Confronted with such evidence 'why do politicians … persist on this track?' (p 1128). Why indeed. But they do, along with their advisers egging them on. As well as being dunces, they are the 'intellectual zombies' to whom Evans (2005) has referred, who repeatedly resurface in health policy discourse.

The concern must be that the public is sleepwalking into an NHS that will be very different from that with which it has been familiar. The brand and logo may stay the same, but increasingly they are a façade behind which a very different, and hollowed-out, NHS is taking shape. As one prominent clinician has stated in somewhat stark terms, the NHS:

> is being dismantled by stealth, cloaked by the rhetoric of 'patient choice'. Instead of money flowing to where it is most needed, it is increasingly flowing to shareholders. Instead of cooperation, we have competition. In place of the invaluable

public sector ethos that has sustained the NHS, we have the
profit motive. (Savage 2006: 3)

These prescient words were written four years ahead of the coalition
government's much criticised and vigorously opposed NHS changes.
Yet very little of substance was abandoned or amended and the
changes remained largely intact and passed into law. The problem, it
seems, is that once the genie is out of the bottle, thanks to the actions
of the Labour governments from 1997 to 2010, it becomes all but
impossible to put it back in again. So, while some commentators believe
that it is time to replace the existing market-based reforms and the
commissioner–provider separation with a different approach, all the
effort and energy in England if not elsewhere in the UK are going in
precisely the opposite direction.

SEVEN

The health debate: what and where next?

Introduction

Health system reform is likely to remain an international preoccupation as countries of different political persuasions and at different stages of development seek to balance rising demand and limited resources. In balancing these, policy makers have to wrestle with a variety of interlocking political cleavages that constitute an ongoing health debate. The spread of universal health coverage, actively encouraged by the World Health Organisation (WHO) and others, is an example of this global phenomenon.

The purpose of this book has been to describe and analyse several of the principal policy cleavages that have exercised, and continue to preoccupy, policy makers in their never-ending pursuit of the perfect health system. On the evidence reviewed here, such a laudable goal is probably unattainable – less imperfection is the best that can be hoped for – although this truism will not prevent policy makers and their advisers from making the attempt, especially in a context where there is a loss of institutional memory and a seeming reluctance to learn from history. As Judt perceptively cautions: 'there is something worse than idealising the past ... forgetting it' (Judt 2010: 41-2).

Running through each of the policy cleavages considered here – the funding and organisation of health systems, the attempt to shift the emphasis from health care to health to combat dramatically rising lifestyle problems like obesity, alcohol misuse and mental ill-health, priority setting and rationing health care, and the appeal of markets and choice and competition as drivers for reform – is a tension between the bureaucratic reformers and market reformers that Alford (1975) described over 30 years ago. It is hard to identify any health issue that is not conceptualised or presented in such terms: with reformers belonging in one camp or the other and often moving back and forth between them. It is probably fair to conclude that in contemporary health policy it is the market reformers who are in the ascendant.

Another long-standing tension in health policy – that between centralisers and decentralisers – can also be presented in terms of those who may be deemed bureaucratic reformers, who favour central control and change led from the top (in the manner of 'Fordist' reformers), and those who are labelled market reformers who subscribe to locally generated, decentralised change (akin to 'post-Fordist' reformers). Perhaps the issue of health care priority setting or rationing is the best example of the centralisation versus decentralisation tension, since the elimination of the so-called postcode lottery when it comes to prescribing treatment may be deemed unacceptable if it is seen to create pressure for uniformity and state-driven national standards of care and treatment that pre-empt a significant degree of local determination. The fact that pressure to devolve responsibility and move away from unbridled state power results in precisely such variations cuts little ice with those puzzled as to why they cannot get access to a drug that is available a few miles away.

Such manifestations of this tension are becoming more frequent in the UK as devolution matures and Wales, Scotland and Northern Ireland increasingly go their separate ways and follow different paths in health policy. In respect of Scotland, the huge political shifts witnessed in recent years favouring independence and a break with the neoliberal policies of the UK government that most Scots have not voted for were not predicted a decade or so ago. Within England, pressures to devolve power and responsibility are also gathering pace following the sudden and rather unexpected announcement of the Greater Manchester Health and Social Care Devolution initiative (Association of Greater Manchester Authorities et al 2015). The Memorandum of Understanding, which has the backing of NHS England and others, sets out an ambitious and challenging agenda designed to encourage the integration of services to improve the health and wellbeing of the

2.8 million citizens of Greater Manchester with a budget of around £6 billion in 2015/16. Full devolution will commence in April 2016 and will provide democratic oversight of NHS services, thereby overcoming the so-called 'democratic deficit' that has long plagued the NHS. The developments occurring in Greater Manchester form the cornerstone of the so-called Northern Powerhouse initiative designed to shift power and resources from the South to the North. They are being followed by other initiatives affecting some other English regions.

Of course, there are risks involved in devolving powers (for a review of some of these, see Buck 2015; Gamsu 2015; Hudson 2015) and it is not even clear how far devolved powers will stick with health ministers declaring that they will retain reserve powers to overturn any decisions made locally (Paine 2015). If these are decisions over which they disapprove, it hardly amounts to a ringing endorsement of the virtues of devolution. Nevertheless, even allowing for possible risks, especially at a time of public spending cuts affecting local government most of all and thereby allowing the government to diffuse blame if things go wrong, the proposals do offer an opportunity of building stronger relationships with communities and possibly challenging the neoliberal embrace of health policy (Local Government Association 2015). Moreover, given the built-in tension between a health service that is national and a level of government that is local, greater local autonomy would come at the expense of a wish to maintain a uniform NHS, although there is no compelling evidence of a desire for growing variation even if it is a likely consequence of many of the government's policies such as choice and competition. It seems to be yet another policy fashion that for a time is in 'good currency' before being replaced by something else.

The market reforms that have swept through the health systems in many countries over the past decade or so can be regarded as another example of policy fashion, although clearly a more enduring one. As described in earlier chapters, they continue to remain in vogue, having briefly lost their allure in the late 1990s. There is an assumption that the faith being placed on markets in health systems will once again ebb and then flow – it is in the nature of health policy and the cyclical nature of fashion that this will be so. And this is because, as Paton explains, the rationale for choice and competition and markets 'is at root political rather than based upon evaluation of health reform' (2006: 130). But there is also a risk that, following Evans' warning about not being able to put the genie back in the bottle, that things will change in a way that cannot be reversed and that health policy will never quite be the same again (Evans 2005).

Following the NHS changes commencing in 2010, enshrined in the Health and Social Care Act 2012, that is the great fear among critics of the changes and defenders of the NHS. You do not have to be a conspiracy theorist to suspect if not a plot then a consensus among the political elite within all parties that choice and competition are here to stay (Pollock 2005 and 2015; Leys and Player 2011; Owen 2014; Davis et al 2015; Jones 2015). The issue is where all this is likely to lead. The NHS chief executive, Simon Stevens, states in *The National Health Service Five Year Forward View* that nothing confronting the NHS 'suggests that continuing with a comprehensive tax-funded NHS is intrinsically un-doable' (NHS England 2014, paragraph 16: 5). On the other hand, critics of recent changes in the NHS fear that in future it will be a state insurance provider and not a state deliverer. This claim was made in 2010 by Mark Britnell, a former head of NHS commissioning who is now head of healthcare in Europe and the UK for the management consultancy KPMG. Of course, both Stevens and Britnell may be correct since, as the last chapter noted, the current government is strongly in favour of outsourcing and actively encouraging private providers to bid for contracts they have been winning. And there is nothing in the new models of care proposed by NHS England and being actively developed in multiple sites to prevent these schemes being run by private providers or by a mix of public-private consortia.

Advocates of market-style incentives rarely acknowledge the drawbacks of such a system and of course that is not their main concern or perhaps motive. Rather it is to further their own interests, as Jones describes in his critique of the establishment and its ruling elites (Jones 2015). The issue has more to do with politics and power than with the effective delivery of services. Nevertheless, it is worth listing some of the more common drawbacks, including those discussed in Chapter Six. They are:

- fragmentation of care as different hospitals and other facilities compete with each other for resources and patients;
- loss of integration and joined-up policy and care as health care services compete with each other for market share;
- lack of a whole-systems approach in prioritising policy around chronic disease and public health;
- inability of governments to manage relationships and confront powerful vested interests;
- high cost of regulation as a result of 'mission creep' that arises in the desperate attempt by government to regulate market behaviour.

As noted in Chapter Two, there are lessons to be learnt from pre-NHS history. However, these appear to have been conveniently ignored, overlooked or selectively chosen to justify particular policies such as the encouragement of social enterprises, which is presented in terms of a return to socialism's roots in the 1920s and the appearance of the cooperative movement. Indeed, paradoxically, and despite its fixation with progress and modernity, the government appears to have embarked upon a course of action that seems destined to recreate much of that history in some form or other – a case of back to the future.

The effects of the latest market changes in the English NHS and in other countries, like the Netherlands, continue to work through the system and are still being felt. Doubtless, there will be adjustments made that might either strengthen or weaken market forces. But it is in assuming that perfect competition will be possible in place of underperforming monopoly public services that advocates of the market are at their most naive. Why this should be so is never satisfactorily explained. Indeed, because the drivers are largely ideological and political, the absence of convincing evidence does not appear to be a concern. At best, what health system change demonstrates is a belief in policy-informed evidence rather than evidence-based policy. The

THE HEALTH DEBATE [SECOND EDITION]

pro-choice advocates either fail to appreciate the political, value-driven and ultimately ideological nature of the debate, in the conduct of which evidence is judiciously deployed to support whatever value position is favoured, or they somewhat nakedly make no pretence of the fact that it is their convictions and beliefs that determine and drive their actions.

Where once opponents of extending markets to, and/or expanding markets in, health systems would have advocated for a genuine alternative model or paradigm, now they rather feebly believe that the battle has been lost and that the only option is to work with such interests in order to ensure that they produce social or public, rather than solely shareholder, value. However, as has been seen in the area of tobacco control or in the operations of the powerful vested interests that make up the food and drink conglomerates, achieving social objectives through attempts at partnership working, via responsibility deals or some other mechanism, is likely to be a difficult road, with progress by no means guaranteed. A fundamental characteristic of markets is that participants do whatever pays best; need, or accommodating the wishes and preferences of politicians and policy makers, is irrelevant. To believe, as some commentators naively do (Appleby 2015), that the perversities and dysfunctional features of markets can be confronted and defeated by a strong and sophisticated regulatory environment, flies in the face of all the evidence (see Chapter Six).

The prevailing orthodoxy in many countries appears to be that as long as the state controls the funding of health care it matters less who provides it. A mixed economy of care is in high fashion as an exemplar of the end of ideology concerning public versus private provision and demonstrating a pragmatic commitment to efficient and effective delivery of care regardless of its source. Bureaucratic reforms and solutions have been found wanting and, so we are led to believe, market-style reforms will succeed where they have failed. But the prognosis is not quite so straightforward for reasons Alford (1975) so ably articulates. His classic study of health care politics warrants careful study for its relevance to contemporary health systems.

A structural perspective on health system reform: revisiting Alford

Alford's central thesis is that reform strategies based on either markets or bureaucratic models are unlikely to succeed because they neglect the way in which groups within health care systems develop vital interests that sustain the present system and vitiate attempts at reform. The two types of reform are not mere ideological constructs:

> [They] are also analyses of the structure of health care which rest upon different empirical assumptions about the nature and power of the health profession, the nature of medical technologies, the role of the hospital, and the role of the patient ... as passively receiving or actively demanding a greater quality and quantity of health care. (Alford 1975: 5)

It is a failure on the part of policy makers to appreciate this feature of both market and bureaucratic reform models that accounts for the disappointment that quickly sets in when reforms do not match expectations.

Alford's 'structural interest' perspective remains critical in understanding the organisational life of health systems regardless of whether they are predisposed to market or bureaucratic ideal types, or some mix of the two. His analysis of these various interests remains fresh and vibrant. According to his essentially political science perspective – a type of analysis that is sadly rare in contemporary social science inquiry (Hunter 2015a and 2015b) – powerful interests benefit from the health system (any health system) precisely as it is. This applies regardless of whether it is a US-style market system or a UK-style national health system. In either model, the 'dominant' interests (clinicians – the 'professional monopolists') manage to do rather nicely and, for all the turbulence associated with health system reforms, exercise considerable power to preserve their privileges. For their part, the challenging interests (managers – the 'corporate rationalisers') are party to a constant expansion of their functions, power and resources justified by the need to control the professional monopolists. Meanwhile, the goals of easily

THE HEALTH DEBATE [SECOND EDITION]

accessible, low-cost and equitable health care remain elusive. With the exception of a health system like Cuba's, it may be possible to achieve one or two of these goals but not all three.

Whether the professional monopolists have begun to see their power base curbed in recent years in the face of the challenge from the corporate rationalisers is a matter for empirical inquiry and the subject of much debate among researchers, as earlier chapters have noted. Certainly, the various reforms of health systems over the years have had, as a common feature, the shifting of the frontier between medicine and management in favour of the latter. There has been a sustained challenge to medicine's hegemony, witnessed most recently in England with the government's determination to introduce seven day working in the NHS accompanied by the introduction of a new contract for junior doctors. The proposed changes have been criticised by the British Medical Association and others and strike action has been threatened if changes are not forthcoming. But it remains to be seen how much remains at the level of rhetoric or symbolic gesturing without seriously affecting the actual working practices of frontline clinicians is hard to determine. This situation serves to emphasise the nature of the dilemma and the paradox at its heart: namely, that while doctors may be perceived as the cause of many of the problems facing health systems, they are also pivotal to their solution. Any alternative to bureaucratic or market reforms ignores this fact at its peril. The new models of care being promoted by NHS England through its Vanguards initiative acknowledge this truth. Their success is crucially dependent on local clinicians and managers leading and driving change. Paradoxically, it seems that Alford's bureaucratic reformers have not been entirely inactive in this regard or been pushed aside by the market reformers who have been in the ascendant. Working with the approach set out in the *National Health Service Five Year Forward View*, the 'bureaucratic reformers' (Alford 1975) are creating the conditions and providing the support for local change to occur by whatever means is deemed appropriate. Only time will tell if this experiment has succeeded or not.

Alford's depiction of the tensions in health system reform as those that are manifest between the dominant and challenging interests only goes to reinforce the powerlessness of the repressed interests – the general public. Belatedly, governments in various countries have begun to talk about the 'expert patient', the patient as 'co-producer', and are seeking to devise ways of giving patients and communities more say not only in how decisions might affect them but also, more importantly, in how those decisions are made in the first place. The language of choice and devolved responsibility and of creating new forms of governance involving local communities in directly owning health care facilities, like foundation hospital trusts in England, and managing them through new mutual forms of organisation, like social enterprises, are examples of how policy makers are looking to make the traditionally repressed interests more powerful in determining the future direction of health systems, especially when it comes to influencing priorities. It is too early to conclude whether such a shift in power will or can occur, or whether the resilience of the dominant interests, to which the challenging interests may well ally themselves, will prevail and frustrate attempts at consciousness raising among the public. However, as was explained in Chapter Five, attempts to engage the public in making rationing decisions have been fraught with problems.

What might drive change and truly empower the public is the acknowledgement that chronic disease is of growing significance as the overall health status of populations improves and people live longer. The management of chronic disease is where the attractions of co-production are at their most powerful and convincing. The challenges from public health, considered in Chapter Three, might also trigger an alternative way of working since tackling them demands a different kind of partnership between public and governments and a stewardship model of governance that puts the promotion and protection of health at the top of what governments exist to do.

Is there another way?

In England, the constant refrain is that there is no alternative to markets (and certainly no desire for a return to outmoded bureaucratic structures) despite the fact that the other three countries making up the UK – Wales, Scotland and Northern Ireland – are actively devising their own distinct approaches to health policy using a vocabulary that makes little or no mention of choice, competition or markets. Maybe they will discover an alternative road map. Indeed, in both Wales and Scotland, there are already detailed road maps. In Wales, the Bevan Commission set up by the Welsh government under Sir Mansel Aylward's chairmanship proposed a future direction based on integrated services informed by improvement science methods derived from research and a plan-do-study-act cycle focused on improvement strategies to ensure services are delivered efficiently and effectively (Aylward 2011).The commission went further and emphasised the need to go against the prevailing trend in many European health systems by asserting that the moral principles underlying collective, planned provision needed to be renewed and rearticulated.

In Scotland, the Scottish government established the Christie Commission on the Future Delivery of Public Services, which also calls for more collaborative working across public services with an emphasis on co-production between those using and those providing services and a renewed focus on prevention and early years interventions to ease pressures downstream on public services (Christie 2011).What is notable about both these road maps is that they eschew the language of choice, competition, markets, outsourcing and privatisation, and seek instead to reaffirm the vital importance of public services by updating the public service ethos supporting them.

But a note of caution is in order. Often the rhetoric is not matched by the reality. For example, in a review of social policy for disabled people in Scotland, the conclusion reached is that to date social care policies for this group 'suggests that a mix of path dependency and policy conservatism (even among political parties committed to social justice) will continue to operate as a significant brake on the pace and scope of any change' (Rummery and McAngus 2015: 238).This is not to argue that another way is not possible, but simply to stress the importance of political leadership in its implementation.We also know from research comparing the performance of the four UK health systems that the market-style changes introduced in England together with the continuous structural changes that have occurred have not resulted in improved performance (Bevan et al 2014).

In considering whether or not there is a better alternative to the current system following the most recent health system changes in England, there is no shortage of proposals for further changes, although the emphasis is on these occurring in a bottom-up rather than a top-down fashion (see, for example, Greener et al 2014). Among these proposed changes are the new care models set out in *The National Health Service Five Year Forward View* (NHS England 2014), collectively known as the Vanguard projects, which have been launched by NHS England (50 so far). Then there are individual budgets, designed to allow certain groups of patients to buy their own care and mix of services as they consider appropriate. These and other similar policies can be viewed as extensions of the increasing marketisation and commodification of health care as witnessed in recent years in many health systems such as the UK NHS. They 'need not do so but could represent an approach to reform predicated on a different set of values and principles at some remove from those that underpinned the NHS when it was born 60 years ago.

At this point, let us return to the main question being posed in this final chapter: is there another way that avoids, on the one hand, retreating into a misplaced, and perhaps nostalgic, faith that all has been well in the NHS in the past – that there may have existed in the mists of time a mythical golden age to which we should return – and, on the other hand, subscribing to a naive yet dangerous and misplaced faith that simply handing health and health care over to the marketplace will somehow achieve the desired high performance and perfect policy that has hitherto eluded health systems and flies in the face of all the evidence? The simple answer is 'yes', although as a preface to exploring what the alternative might look like, there is a prior need to acknowledge 'the essential rationale of public service' and draw a distinction between the public service orientation on the one hand and consumerism on the other hand that is the hallmark of markets (Clarke and Stewart 1988).

Rediscovering public service

It is important to remember, despite being unfashionable to do so, that services like health have been placed in the public sector precisely because they are different from those in the private sector and demand to be run as such. This point is not lost on members of the public or service users. As Catherine Needham argues in her study of public service reform under New Labour, far from expecting public services to become more like the private sector, the public 'want them to be more like what they felt public services should be' (Needham 2008a: 194). Such a response is strikingly at odds with successive governments insistence that choice is what people want. Such evidence as exists does not bear that out, as we saw in Chapter Six. In general, people have not exercised a choice to go to alternatives to local providers.

Similarly, the adoption of a particular type of business management derived from Fordist or new public management (NPM) thinking is deeply flawed when it comes to asserting the distinctiveness of public services. Here, considerations determined by the political process or marketplace, rather than considerations of the economic marketplace, are critical. For these reasons, new public management's assumption that there are universal ways of managing is misguided and even disingenuous (Stewart 1998). In the public domain, management 'has to be grounded in the distinctive purposes of the public domain which political theory would suggest involve democracy, community, citizenship, equity, and discourse' (Stewart 1998: 23). Meek (2014: 250) makes a similar point when he writes about entities that are fundamentally unlike competing private firms 'that can't ... be deemed naturally 'private industries' or 'public industries' but can only be considered political industries'.

Management in the public domain must also recognise that there are 'distinctive tasks such as balancing values and interests and the exercise of legitimised coercion' (Stewart 1998: 23). Judgement is seen as critical and yet has been neglected in management studies and virtually driven out altogether by NPM and its grip on the public service reform agenda. NPM, as we saw in Chapter Four, is itself a spin-off from the preoccupation with market models of reform and management principles and practices borrowed from the business sector. Judgement is difficult, but, as Stewart argues, quoting Walsh, 'the public realm deals with the sort of services that cannot be delivered without discretion at the point of implementation and delivery, and choice at the political level, both of which demand good judgement' (Stewart 1998: 24). Indeed, managing in the public domain requires the exercise of political judgement since the public interest can never be finally defined – it is constantly being renegotiated as circumstances change.

What amounts to an erosion of the public realm lies at the heart of Judt's critique of private affluence and public squalor (Judt 2010). The UK is witnessing among the greatest extremes of private privilege and public indifference, with a resulting increase in inequality. This has a direct impact on public services like the NHS, as we saw in Chapter Three. As a result of a dismantling of the welfare state, 'the UK is now more unequal – in incomes, wealth, health, education and life chances – than at any time since the 1920s' (Judt 2010: 14).

Sandel makes a similar point when he argues that markets and the commodification of public services erode commonality (Sandel 2013). He continues: 'the marketization of everything means that people of affluence and people of modest means lead increasingly separate lives' (Sandel 2013: 203). This cannot be good for democracy and yet it is happening without public debate and in the midst of public indifference. It is an example of what Judt terms 'the unbearable lightness of politics' (Judt 2010: 81). Instead of being viewed as solutions to many of society's complex problems, including health, government and politics are seen as the problem. In their place, the 'cult of the private' and the worship of the private sector go unchecked and remain unaccountable. That these choices are in fact intensely political seems to have escaped an ever-sceptical if not cynical public. Public indifference can be tolerated in the short term, but its long-term consequences are corrosive. And yet if we are to challenge the prevailing stubborn orthodoxy, we need to become politically mobilised, rediscovering the public realm and arresting, if not reversing, the disintegration of the public sector. In fact, we need to re-politicise public policy in order to bring about change and improvement (Pfeffer 1992). Unless the political determinants of health are appreciated, the illusion that technical fixes exist for health problems will prevail.

As we saw in Chapter Five in a review of health care rationing and priority setting, the science of evidence-based medicine is imperfect and does not obviate or pre-empt the need for judgement that has to be exercised in particular contexts and rightly so (Greenhalgh et al 2014). Universal prescriptions of the type favoured by rational rationers are simply unrealistic and will not work. 'Political judgement involves balancing values and interests and that requires understanding of those values and interests' (Stewart 1998: 24).

Such concerns are not confined to the NHS or the UK. Similar debates are to be heard in New Zealand, where the weaknesses of a market approach, a route the country travelled with even greater vigour and conviction than the UK did back in the early 1990s, have been analysed by Ian Powell, executive director of the Association of Salaried Medical Specialists. For Powell, hankering after market solutions omits any mention of why public health systems developed in the first place. In a lecture delivered in July 2006, he said:

> If the objective is to produce a universally available and comprehensive public good then an integrated and co-ordinated system is necessary rather than a reliance on a system more orientated towards niche markets and profits. It requires a high level of public funding and benefits from a high level of public provision. Private systems cannot do this because it is not their reason for being. (Powell 2005)

Powell also makes the point that competitive tendering and other market-type mechanisms will increase transaction and bureaucratic costs, increase fragmentation between services, risk destabilising planning for service delivery in public facilities, and work contrary to collaborative partnerships over service organisation and delivery.

Such legitimate concerns and risks serve as important reminders and parameters within which to consider an alternative approach to reform in the NHS, which remains committed to a public service ethos or orientation. What is needed, and is arguably largely missing from the current debate about health and health care, is a reconceptualisation of what it means to provide a public service in the 21st century and the nature of professionalism in this endeavour. Attempts are being made to define a third way between old-style public services on the one hand and free market provision on the other. Such attempts take the form of encouraging the emergence of a range of not-for-profit organisations collectively known as social enterprises, public interest companies, mutuals, cooperatives and suchlike. As noted earlier, many New Labour reformers see nothing incompatible between such models and the calls in the 1920s from the guild socialists for such community-based organisational forms to flourish, although such an interpretation of history may not be wholly accurate (Gorsky 2006).

When NHS foundation trusts were first established, they were described as new organisational forms that would allow their ownership to reside with local communities. Few now hold this view and, as we noted in Chapter Six, their future is in some doubt. Moreover, when judged against for-profit business criteria, not-for-profit organisations quickly begin to look indistinguishable from such entities (Marks and Hunter 2007). In any event, while much is made of the need to involve the public in running public organisations and often technically complex services like hospitals, is there a significant hunger among the public for taking these into their direct control? Who has the time to devote to such tasks in anything other than a purely nominal or tokenistic way? How realistic is it to expect social enterprises to take over and run vast swaths of local services in ways that are both equitable and adhere to agreed minimum standards? Is there a risk that the cost of regulating such a diverse marketplace becomes prohibitive and ends up stultifying the very innovation and creativity that is being sought? There may well be a place for new models of public ownership, especially in some areas of chronic care, but the more likely reality is that after a while people will tire of owning/running services, with the likely consequence that the services will pass into private ownership and control of a very different nature.

Renewing professionalism: the potential of co-production

Perhaps there is another way that builds on the systems and traditions already established in health service organisations such as the NHS but which recent changes have for whatever reason chosen to ignore. Before jettisoning, or abandoning altogether – if it is not already too late – the structures, systems and patterns of behaviour that have evolved over the life of the NHS, policy makers could consider devoting greater attention to how they might be reconfigured or redirected without resorting to wholesale structural changes and market-style lures that bring with them their own problems, perversities and risks – a case, perhaps, of the cure killing the patient. Such an alternative 'third way' might be based on three particular dimensions:

- clinical governance as a development tool;
- re-engagement of clinicians as co-producers;
- responsible autonomy.

Few informed observers doubt that the NHS requires a modified conception of public service to fit it for the challenges of the 21st century. Such a shift is necessary to embrace notions of public participation through citizenship, and a refreshed or renewed conception of professionalism best described as 'responsible professionalism'. As part of these developments, there needs to be effective co-production of health between the public and professions, one that is based not on consumer–producer relationships in adversarial terms but on highlighting their interdependence in a system of negotiated order. There is no place in such arrangements for a return to professional dominance or paternalism – a charge all too easily though unfairly levelled at many critics of the market-style reforms. Indeed, as was discussed in Chapter Four, in diagnosing the deficiencies and flaws in the NHS there was widespread agreement across the political spectrum with the thrust of New Labour's analysis.

Ardent supporters of the NHS, including those of a socialist persuasion such as Julian Tudor Hart (1994), are among the fiercest critics of the professional abuse of power in health systems as well as being staunch advocates of patients as co-producers of health. 'Recognition of patients as co-producers rather than consumers would begin to solve several problems which are otherwise likely to get worse. As co-producers, patients must share much more actively both in defining their problems and in devising feasible solutions, than they have in the past' (Tudor Hart 1994: 43). For Tudor Hart, this model of co-production is 'a different, socialist way to look at health production in the NHS, as neither a state funded autonomous medical hierarchy nor a market of competing corporations dominated by business-trained executives' (1994: 43). The challenge is taken up by Catherine Needham, who argues that in a co-productive model, 'staff on the frontline of public services are recognised to have a distinctive voice and expertise as a result of regular interaction with service users' (2008b: 222). The co-productive approach is a challenge to Fordist and NPM concepts of how to improve public services and has much more in common with notions of systems thinking and of how complex adaptive systems function.

For example, organisational psychologist John Seddon (2003) advocates ending the tyranny of targets, which he believes only serve to foster compliance rather than innovation. It is not a case of having fewer or better targets, as some critics of the current system of top-down imposed targets propose, a variant that Seddon believes misses the point, namely that managing by targets in any shape or form is dysfunctional, especially when the targets are divorced from the people who are expected to deliver them. In place of targets, Seddon proposes that public sector organisations should be required to establish measures that, in their view, help them understand and improve performance. Upon inspection, they would be required to demonstrate how they have satisfied the requirement and to what effect. The principal advantage of such an approach is that it places the locus of control where it needs to belong: locally, with those on the front line. A possible drawback is that inspection and regulation bring with them their own problems and as the Mid Staffordshire scandal demonstrated, they are not infallible (Francis 2013).

In many health systems, including the British NHS, such an approach demands a new working relationship between clinicians (a term used to include doctors and nurses) and managers (Hunter et al 2014). Above all, it requires clinicians to be at the centre of the management task. Roy Griffiths, the architect of general management in the NHS, introduced in 1983, maintained that doctors were the 'natural managers'. But instead of going with the grain and working with this reality, government-led health policy has ignored such critical dynamics. The result has been an unhealthy stand-off between these two tribes (clinicians and managers), which has come to act as a major fault line. It has been always present in the NHS since its inception but it is now in danger of becoming active. Every reorganisation to date has only succeeded in making the situation between these tribes worse and more antagonistic. As long as clinicians exercise power without responsibility, the NHS will fail to improve on the scale necessary. It then becomes an easy target to blame for all resulting woes and ills, many of which beset any health system to some degree regardless of its funding or organisation.

Clinical governance may represent the key to redefining the relationship between clinicians and managers. But if it is to mean anything other than fine sentiments, it has to be linked to structures and processes that integrate financial control, service performance and clinical quality in ways that will both engage clinicians and generate service improvements. Furthermore, only through such means can 'responsible autonomy' be re-established as a founding principle in the performance and organisation of clinical work. The focus by Degeling and his colleagues on clinical governance as a development tool is critical to the systematisation of clinical work proposed (Degeling at al 2004). It requires the implementation of a model that, first, is based on the centrality of clinician involvement in the design, provision and improvement of care; and, second, is structured to change how clinical work is conceived, organised and performed. For such a model to be meaningful, clarity is required about what can and needs to be done at service delivery levels to encourage and support doctors, nurses, allied health workers and managers to adopt new ways of working that:

- accept interconnections between clinical and resource dimensions of care;
- recognise the need to balance clinical autonomy with transparent accountability;
- support the systematisation of clinical work and bring it within the ambit of process control;
- subscribe to the power-sharing implications of more integrated and team-based approaches to clinical work performance and evaluation.

It may well be that system redesign and management action to engage clinicians can bring health system objectives closer to those of society. Many observers consider that such a road map would be a more fruitful one to follow than a reliance on competitive markets (Smith 2003). Indeed, Smith claims it is difficult to see how the introduction of a competitive market into health and health care will help it move towards a more effective and engaged professional culture. Precisely the opposite could occur, with the encouragement of competitive behaviour adversely affecting professional willingness to share experience and undertake activities that lie outside agreed contractual requirements. The consequence could be fragmented and disintegrated services at a time when a whole-systems approach and integrated care are desired.

None of what is being suggested here is especially novel or outlandish. Elements can be identified somewhere in the NHS and have much in common with the systems approach favoured by Seddon and by other analysts who have written about 'wicked problems' in public policy (Australian Government and Australian Public Service Commission 2007), and complexity and complex adaptive systems (see, for example, Plsek and Greenhalgh 2001; Chapman 2004; De Savigny and Adam 2009). Yet it has not happened in a consistent or systematised way or on a scale sufficient to amount to a tipping point or paradigm shift. The tragedy and missed opportunity is that, as noted in Chapter Four, many of New Labour's early reforms were welcome and did appear to understand and appreciate these systemic issues. But for whatever reason, perhaps the ineptitude of politicians as managers being a major cause, there was insufficient and ineffective follow-through. The reform agenda was hijacked, on the basis of little evidence that it would work, by a focus on structures, targets, and a seductive belief that markets, with their focus on choice and competition, held the answers. Whatever the explanation, Labour's later reforms coupled with those introduced by the coalition government between 2010 and 2015 have amounted to a cruel distraction from grappling with the managerial and professional conundrum that has prevailed in the NHS over its lifespan (Hunter 2006a).

There is also a risk that introducing the shift in approach outlined above as an alternative to choice and competition is likely to be dismissed as yet another passing management fad (Degeling et al 2001). Health care staff, already cynical, demoralised and weary from reorganisation fatigue, may view the new approach with considerable scepticism, and it could exacerbate the climate of distrust that already permeates relations between clinical and management staff. However, what is known from a record of health care reform stretching back over more than 30 years in the UK is that top-down reform initiatives imposed on a highly professionalised workforce by a hierarchical authority are destined to fail. Critical to securing sustainable change is the realisation noted earlier that while clinicians may be part of the problem, they are also central to its solution. This is not a lament for a return to some mythical Eden when clinicians were left to their own devices and remained largely unaccountable for their actions. But just as producer dominance is a danger to be avoided, so also is a deliberate attempt to ignore or bypass producers' knowledge and experience altogether. To his credit, the NHS chief executive, Simon Stevens, appears to acknowledge this concern and is keen for clinicians working with managers to lead the system changes he believes are essential to transform the NHS and render it fit for the challenges it faces (NHS England 2014). But to his critics, Stevens is regarded with intense suspicion as the enemy within following his spell with the US private health insurance company, United Health. Those tracking his career and public utterances suspect him of being a Trojan Horse in the midst of the NHS intent on opening it up to private sector interests.

On the other side, Stevens' defenders choose to emphasise his public sector credentials and insist that he did not return to the UK from the US to preside over the NHS's demise. Only time will tell who is right.

Regardless of what ultimately happens in respect of the new models of care being developed, there is an important issue at stake concerning the craftsmanship that lies at the core of sound professional practice. Craftsmanship is not something that can be taught along the lines of painting by numbers. It requires years of experience to acquire the exercise of judgement and tacit knowledge that only experience can bring. The quality of health care will ultimately always depend on professional judgement that 'cannot be regulated, audited or commercialised away without services deteriorating' (Lawson 2007: 40). The idea of clinical 'craft' is demeaned by such notions and by the managerial revolution that has swept through health care since the 1970s but with a growing intensity through the past decade or so (Sennett 2008). According to Sennett, 'to do good work means to be curious about, to investigate, and to learn from ambiguity' (2008: 48). Furthermore, he observes that craft quality emerges from the importance of tacit knowledge and habits and writes: 'When an institution like the NHS, in churning reform, doesn't allow the tacit anchor to develop, then the motor of judgement stalls. People have no experience to judge, just a set of abstract propositions about good-quality work' (Sennett 2008: 50). The failure in government health policy in recent years has been a misconceived desire 'to root out embedded knowledge' and 'expose it to the cleansing of rational analysis' while becoming frustrated over the recognition that much tacit knowledge is precisely the thing that cannot be 'put into words' or rendered 'as logical propositions' (Sennett 2008: 51).

The danger becomes one of placing too much emphasis and faith on meeting targets imposed on professionals who may not subscribe to or, in the jargon, 'own' them. Or there may be opposition to the approach in general for the reasons articulated by critics like Seddon. As was noted in Chapter Four, a target-based approach risks diverting energies and talent to meeting targets (the phenomenon of managing to target) rather than to achieving the core purpose of the NHS, namely, the prevention and treatment of disease, which most observers, including unusually the NHS chief executive, acknowledge. Moreover, the manner in which targets have been imposed and performance managed has tended to favour acute care services. Preventing ill-health, as was pointed out in Chapter Three, has not received the attention it should, given the priority ostensibly accorded it by the government.

The embodiment of true craftsmanship, as defined by Sennett, demands a constant interplay between tacit knowledge and explicit awareness or critique. This tension posits that muddling through or doing a job that is just good enough is not sufficient and that experience needs to be combined with a systematic or standardised approach where that is possible and desirable. There is room in health care, therefore, for management approaches such as lean thinking and other improvement science methods, which may be applied to areas of care that can be subject to, and benefit from, systematisation (for an evaluation of such an approach applied to a whole English region – the North East Transformation System [NETS] – see Hunter et al 2014). They should be used to free up professionals to exercise judgement and draw on tacit knowledge where required and not employed to obliterate or replace these qualities of craftsmanship. However, what our study of transformational change revealed was that complex systems change demands time and stability. Paradoxically, there has to be a freezing of the organisation in order to change it effectively. Structures that are in the midst of change and staff churn are not well placed to undertake or sustain cultural change of the type that underpinned NETS. And so it proved. A study of NETS showed that the initiative, despite achieving much positive change, was ultimately derailed by the coalition government's NHS changes introduced in 2010 (Hunter et al 2015). The finding was not especially novel or unexpected, but policy makers ignore such insights at their peril (except that policy makers probably do not care that much since they are driven not by evidence of what works but by their own beliefs and interests). If there is to be another way, the political dimension of policy making has to be understood and redirected. We return to this point in the last section below.

The stewardship model of governance

Considerable mention has been made of the shift in policy from health care to health – a shift underway in many health systems as chronic care rises up the policy agenda having overtaken infectious diseases as the principal cause of ill-health. A conundrum for policy makers is how far the thrust of contemporary health policy reform, with its bias towards markets, choice, competition and individualism, is compatible with the need for a focus in broader health policy on stewardship and citizenship in tackling the so-called diseases of comfort or excess (Nuffield Council on Bioethics 2007). Even former government adviser Julian Le Grand, an ardent enthusiast of individual choice in acute health care, acknowledges the limits of such an approach when it comes to public health and the need for state intervention even where it might infringe individual autonomy. The trick, he suggests, is to achieve the ends sought by policy makers by still preserving individual autonomy and avoiding creating a nanny state by the adoption of a libertarian paternalism derived from behavioural economics. The 'nudge' architecture underpinning the new behavioural economics focuses not on denying people choices but on incentivising them to make healthier ones (Thaler and Sunstein 2008).

In its report on ethical issues in public health, the Nuffield Council on Bioethics (2007) goes further and asserts that public health is not generally concerned with the individual but with the population. This means that it is not always easy or appropriate to apply concepts such as autonomy or individual rights. Instead, it adopts the stewardship model (see Box 7.1). The concept of stewardship is intended to convey the idea that liberal states have a duty to protect the needs of people both individually and collectively. It has been defined as 'the careful and responsible management of the well-being of the population' and as constituting 'the very essence of good government' (World Health Organisation 2000). Therefore, stewardship is one of the core functions of the health system (Travis et al 2002). Governments are obliged to ensure the existence of conditions that reduce health inequalities and allow people to be healthy. In its use of the term, WHO views stewardship in respect of health as a key task of government, as it regards good health as a primary asset of a country. There is a hard-nosed argument here since, as was noted in Chapter Three, higher levels of health are associated with improved wellbeing and higher productivity. Stewardship is also an intensely political activity because the way in which it is performed and the goals it pursues, either implicitly or explicitly, involve paying attention to particular values and ignoring, or paying less attention to, others (Hunter et al 2005).

Box 7.1: The stewardship model

Acceptable public health goals include:

- reducing the risks of ill-health that people are exposed to as a result of other people's actions or behaviours;
- reducing causes of ill-health relating to environmental conditions;
- protecting and promoting the health of children and other vulnerable groups;
- helping people to overcome addictions and other unhealthy behaviours;
- ensuring that it is easy for people to lead a healthy life;
- ensuring that people have appropriate access to medical services;
- reducing health inequalities.

Source: Adapted from Nuffield Council on Bioethics (2007).

Through the device of a proposed 'intervention ladder', the Nuffield Council on Bioethics offers a means of thinking about the acceptability and justification of different public health policies (see Box 7.2).

Box 7.2: Intervention ladder

- Eliminate choice;
- restrict choice;
- guide choice through disincentives;
- guide choices through incentives;
- guide choices through changing the default policy;
- enable choice;
- provide information;
- do nothing or simply monitor the current situation.

Source: Nuffield Council on Bioethics (2007).

The least intrusive intervention is non-intervention: to do nothing or at most monitor the situation as a form of 'watchful waiting'. At the other extreme, the most intrusive intervention is to legislate in such a way as to restrict the liberties of individuals, the population as a whole or specific industries. So, for example, eliminating choice might be justified in an infectious disease outbreak where patients have to be compulsorily isolated. Restricted choice might be justified in the attack on obesity and health-related diseases by removing unhealthy ingredients from foods though reformulation, or reducing portion size in restaurants and other food outlets. Or, instead of chips being offered as standard and a salad as an option, the reverse might apply, so that the salad option became standard with chips offered as an option. Various incentives might also be introduced to guide behaviour, such as increasing the price of alcohol and cigarettes and discouraging car use in inner cities. Such an intervention ladder offers a means of assessing the level of government action required in regard to a specific public health challenge. The fact that such measures are being openly discussed offers the prospect of substantive change. It could be that the positive experience of the ban on smoking in public places has encouraged policy makers to be bolder in respect of other public health challenges that are at least as great although as the discussion of obesity policy in Chapter 3 showed, the government has so far resisted taking strong action. True to form, governments are sensitive to the charge of being a nanny state. Yet, is there not a double standard at work here? On the one hand it seems to be acceptable for governments to behave like nanny when it comes to national security issues, including moves to snoop on private citizens' emails and mobile phone calls. On the other hand, when it is a case of how people choose to lead their lives in other domains even though such behaviour has implications for public services like health care and their resourcing, there is a marked reluctance to intervene and excuses are found for not doing so or, as in the case of the smoking ban in public places in England, doing so somewhat reluctantly.

Last word

The founding father of the UK's NHS, Aneuran Bevan, wrote in 1952 that the NHS represented '… a triumphant example of the superiority of collective action and public initiative applied to a segment of society where commercial principles are seen at their worst' (1978: 8). Yet, the direction of health policy over the past decade or so seems intent on introducing, or to be more precise reintroducing, those very same commercial principles, spurred on by a 'progressive' myth that society has changed irreversibly and that there is no other way. This is a political standpoint that has no firm or uncontested basis in the evidence. At the same time, it is not good enough to assert that the NHS in its pre-1974 form, or whatever other date is chosen following the first of many disastrous reorganisations since then, is what we should be aspiring to. A weakness of many of the well-meaning critics of market-style changes to be found in campaigning bodies like Keep Our NHS Public (KONP) is the assumption, often unstated, that the NHS as it was is somehow above criticism (for a good example of KONP's critique, see Davis et al 2015). It is not, and such a view of the NHS verges on the nostalgic and romantic and is unhelpful in addressing its weaknesses. These need to be confronted head on and not lost in the otherwise justified assault on the market-style reforms that have done so much to weaken and undermine the NHS as a noble endeavour.

At issue is the nature and type of change, not the fact of the need for change per se. Arguably, the NHS's tragedy has been its subjugation to so much change of the wrong type, which has made the forces of resistance hostile to change of any type. And who can blame them, given what the workforce has been through and had to endure for the past two decades and more?

There is another way, but only if the public wants it and if policy makers choose to follow it. The fact that they have hitherto decided not to reveals more about the power of those interests driving policy than about the correctness or validity of the prevailing policy. Resorting to the evidence base is no defence because, as has been argued, the evidence for the most part is inconclusive, contested, selectively cited in support of almost any position or simply lacking. And even where it is robust or raises legitimate concerns about the likely impact of a policy, a strongly held ideology will always trump evidence. Evidence-informed policy has its place but can never be the main driver of policy or health reform. Nor should it be. Policy makers have chosen to surround themselves with a particular group of like-minded advisers and consultants who seem to have attended the same pro-marketisation and pro-choice and competition finishing school and who seem to have no real understanding of how complex systems operate or should be managed. But it would be entirely possible for these same policy makers, if they so chose, to turn to a different group of advisers with different ideals, values and capabilities. In the never-ending cut and thrust of politics and power in health policy, perhaps they will or at least be persuaded to do so. Provided, that is, it is not too late. The Canadians have chosen such a break with the past having elected a Liberal government in October 2015 committed to growth and public infrastructure investment in place of a Conservative government wedded to austerity over the past 10 years or so.

Given the events that have occurred between the first and second editions of this book, it may already be too late following the processes and systems put in train and an entrenched set of political interests that have become further entrenched since the UK general election in May 2015. A key theme running through all the policy cleavages explored in this book is the role and place of politics. Understanding the political nature of the policy process is central to any attempt to change direction. Politics is at the heart of all that happens in public policy and in complex systems, like health, with their multiple objectives, levels of decision making and myriad groups of practitioners conducting endless power plays. Making sense of health policy requires understanding the frameworks and beliefs underlying policy makers' choices and the interests they represent, since it is these and not some spurious scientism or notion of evidence that is shaping and driving their choices. But if we are to engage with these issues in a meaningful way that results in change, we need a new and different kind of politics. Judt (2010) refers to 'the unbearable lightness of politics' and to the current generation of political leaders, who 'convey neither conviction or authority', who 'stand for nothing in particular' and who are 'politicians-lite' (Judt 2010: 133-4).

We must do better than this. We know that neoliberalism kills (Mooney 2012; Stuckler and Basu 2013; Schrecker and Bambra 2015). To counter it, we need a new political economy of health that puts politics at the heart of a public debate that is long overdue. In short, we urgently need a health debate.

Postscript

At the time of checking the proofs for this second edition, Jeremy Corbyn was unexpectedly elected the new leader of the Labour Party with an unprecedented mandate from grass-roots members and supporters across the age spectrum. A consequence has been a new energy and feeling of hope that had all but been expunged from the Labour Party. Perhaps my call above that we must do better than this when it comes to the fate of the NHS, and health policy more generally, has been heeded sooner than I expected. Of course it may all end in tears, given the huge odds facing Corbyn and his team, not least those within his own party who wish him gone, but for now he offers hope to those who have felt betrayed by the Labour Party and who yearn for a political vehicle to reflect and advance their concerns.

Let that health debate proceed with renewed vigour and hold out the prospect of change which addresses many of the cleavages reviewed in this book in new and different ways, and from a political perspective rather than in spurious technocratic and managerial ways which simply reinforce those dilemmas and deny their political origins and essential nature.

References

Alford RR (1975) *Health Care Politics*. Chicago, IL: Chicago University Press.

Antonovsky A (1987) *Unravelling the Mystery of Health: how people manage stress and stay well*. San Francisco, CA: Jossey-Bass.

Appleby J (2015) Paid for by the NHS, treated privately, *British Medical Journal*, 350: h3109.

Arrow K (1963) Uncertainty and the welfare economics of medical care, *American Economic Review* 53: 941–73.

Association of Greater Manchester Authorities, NHS England and NHS Greater Manchester Association of Clinical Commissioning Groups (2015) *Greater Manchester Health and Social Care Devolution. Memorandum of Understanding*. Manchester: Association of Greater Manchester Authorities.

Audit Commission (2006) *Early Lessons in Implementing Practice Based Commissioning*. London: Audit Commission.

Audit Commission (2007) *Putting Commissioning into Practice*. London: Audit Commission.

Australian Government and Australian Public Service Commission (2007) *Tackling Wicked Problems: a public policy perspective*. Canberra: Australian Public Service Commission.

Aylward M (2011) *2008-2011 NHS Wales: forging a better future*. Cardiff: Bevan Commission.

Baggott R (2004) *Health and Health Care in Britain*. 3rd edition. Basingstoke: Palgrave.

Baggott R (2007) *Understanding Health Policy*. Bristol: The Policy Press.

Bambra C, Smith KE, Garthwaite K, Joyce K and Hunter D (2011) A labour of Sisyphus? Public policy and health inequalities research from the Black and Acheson reports to the Marmot review, *Journal of Epidemiology and Community Health* 65 (55): 399-406.

Barr DA, Fenton L and Blane D (2008) The claim for patient choice and equity, *Journal of Medical Ethics* 34: 271–4.

Beecham J (2006) *Beyond Boundaries: review of local service delivery* (Beecham Report). Cardiff: Welsh Assembly Government.

Beresford P (2008) Individual budgets could weaken the NHS, *SocietyGuardian* 16 April: 4.

Berridge V (2007) *History Matters? History's role in health policymaking. A research report for History & Policy*. London: Centre for History in Public Health and LSHTM.

Berwick D (2002) Public performance reports and the will for change, *Journal of the American Medical Association* 288 (12): 1523–4.

Bevan A (1978) *In Place of Fear*. London: Quartet Books.

Bevan G and Hood C (2006) What's measured is what matters: targets and gaming in the English public health care system, *Public Administration* 84 (3): 517–38.

Bevan G, Karanikolos M, Exley J, Nolte E, Connolly S and Mays N (2014) *The Four Health Systems of the UK: how do they compare?* London: The Nuffield Trust.

Birt C (2007) *A CAP on Health? The impact of the EU common agricultural policy on public health.* London: Faculty of Public Health.

Blackler F (2006) Chief executives and the modernization of the English National Health Service, *Leadership* 2 (1): 5–30.

Blair T (2006) Speech on healthy lifestyles. 26 July. Nottingham. www.pm.gov.uk

Blank RH and Burau V (2004) *Comparative Health Policy*. London: Palgrave Macmillan.

Bobbitt P (2003) *The Shield of Achilles: war, peace and the course of history*. London: Penguin Books.

Borzaga C and Defourny J (eds) (2001) *The Emergence of Social Enterprise*. London: Routledge.

Boyle S (2011) United Kingdom (England) health system review, *Health Systems in Transition* 13 (1): 1-486.

Braithwaite J, Westbrook MT, Hindle D and Iedema RA (2008) Hospital sector organisational restructuring: evidence of its futility In: McKee L, Ferlie E and Hyde P (eds) *Organising and Reorganising: power and change in health care organisations.* Basingstoke: Palgrave Macmillan.

Bristol Royal Infirmary Inquiry (2001) *Learning from Bristol: the report of the Public Inquiry into Children's Heart Surgery at the Bristol Royal Infirmary 1984–1995*, Cm 5207 (Chairman: Ian Kennedy). London: The Stationery Office.

BMA (British Medical Association) (1995) *Rationing Revisited: a discussion paper.* Health Policy and Economic Research Unit Discussion Paper No 4. London: BMA.

BMA (2007) *A Rational Way Forward for the NHS in England: a discussion paper outlining an alternative approach to health reform.* London: British Medical Association. www.bma.org.uk/ap.nsf/Content/rationalwayforward.

Brown G (2004) *A Modern Agenda for Prosperity and Social Reform.* London: Social Market Foundation.

Brown G (2008) Speech on the National Health Service, 7 January. www.pm.gov.uk.

Bryden A, Petticrew M, Mays N, Eastmure E and Knai C (2013) Voluntary agreements between government and business – a scoping review of the literature with specific reference to the public health responsibility deal, *Health Policy* 110 (2-3): 186-197.

Buck D (2015) Early wins and longer term spadework. In: Local Government Association *Devo Next: English Devolution: local solutions for a healthy nation.* London: LGA: 12-13.

Buck D and Frosini G (2012) *Clustering of Unhealthy Behaviours Over Time.* London: The King's Fund.

Burns H (2015) Health inequalities – why so little progress? *Public Health* 129 (7): 859–53.

Butland B, Jebb S, Kopelman P, McPherson K, Thomas S, Mardell J and Parry V (2007) *Tackling Obesities: Future Choices – Project report, Commissioned by the UK Government's Foresight Programme, Government Office for Science.* London: Department of Innovation, Universities and Skills.

Cabinet Office (2007) *Capability Review of the Department of Health.* London: Cabinet Office.

Centre for Health and the Public Interest (2015) *The Contracting NHS – can the NHS handle the outsourcing of clinical services.* London: Centre for Health and the Public Interest.

Chapman J (2004) *System Failure: why governments must learn to think differently.* 2nd edition. London: Demos.

Charlesworth A (2015) NHS *Finances – the challenge all political parties need to face.* Briefing. London: The Health Foundation.

Chernichovsky D (1995) Health system reforms in industrialised democracies: an emerging paradigm, *Milbank Quarterly* 73 (3): 339–56.

Christensen T and Laegreid P (2007) The whole-of-government approach to public sector reform, *Public Administration Review* 67 (6): 1059–66.

Christie C (2011) *Commission on the Future Delivery of Public Services.* Edinburgh: Scottish Government.

Choi BCK, Hunter DJ, Tsou W and Sainsbury P (2005) Diseases of comfort: primary cause of death in the 22nd century, *Journal of Epidemiology & Community Health* 59: 1030–4.

Clarke J, Newman J and Westmorland L (2008) The antagonisms of choice: New Labour and the reform of public services, *Social Policy & Society* 7(2): 245–53.

Clarke M and Stewart J (1988) *The Enabling Council.* London: Local Government Training Board.

Claxton K (2015) The UK's Cancer Drugs Fund does more harm than good, *New Scientist* 13 January.

Coast J (1997) Rationing within the NHS should be explicit: the case against, *British Medical Journal* 31: 1118–22.

Commission on Social Determinants of Health (2007) *Achieving Health Equity: from root causes to fair outcomes.* Geneva: WHO.

Commission on Social Determinants of Health (2008) *Closing the gap in a generation: health equity through action on the social determinants of health.* Report. Geneva: WHO.

Connolly S, Bevan G and Mays N (2010) *Funding and Performance of Healthcare systems in the Four Countries of the UK Before and After Devolution.* London: The Nuffield Trust.

Cooke G and Lawton K (2008) *Working Out of Poverty: a study of the low paid and the working poor.* London: Institute for Public Policy Research.

Cooper Z and Le Grand J (2007) Choice, competition and the political left, *Eurohealth* 13 (4): 18–20.

Coote A and Hunter DJ (1996) *New Agenda for Health.* London: Institute for Public Policy Research.

Coote A and Penny J (2014) *The Wrong Medicine: a review of the impacts of NHS reforms in England.* London: New Economics Foundation.

Coppard P (2010) Public health as a local government function, *Perspectives on Public Health Series.* London: Local Government Association. www.lgyh.gov.uk/dnlds/Public%20Health%20 as%20a%20Local%20Government%20Function%20-%20Phil%20 Coppard.pdf.

Coulter A and Ham C (eds) (2000) *The Global Challenge of Health Care Rationing.* Buckingham: Open University Press.

Council of the European Union (2006) *2767th Employment, Social Policy, Health and Consumer Affairs Council Meeting. Council Conclusions on Health in All Policies (HiAP)*, 30 November – 1 December, Brussels.

Craig D (2006) *Plundering the Public Sector.* London: Constable.

Daniels N (2000) Accountability for reasonableness, *British Medical Journal* 321: 1300–1.

Davis J, Lister J and Wrigley D (2015) *NHS For Sale: myths, lies and deception.* London: Merlin Press.

Davis K, Stremikis K, Squires D and Schoen C (2014) *Mirror, Mirror on the Wall: how the performance of the US health care system compares internationally. 2014 Update.* New York, NY: The Commonwealth Fund.

Davis K, Schoen C, Schoenbaum SC, Doty MM, Holmgren AL, Kriss JL and Shea KK (2007) *Mirror, Mirror on the Wall: an international update on the comparative performance of American health care.* New York, NY: The Commonwealth Fund.

Dawson S and Dargie C (2002) New public management: a discussion with special reference to UK health. In: McLaughlin K, Osborne SP and Ferlie E (eds) *New Public Management: current trends and future prospects.* London: Routledge.

Degeling P, Kennedy J and Hill M (1998) Do professional subcultures set limits to hospital reform?, *Clinician in Management* 5 (2): 64–9.

Degeling P, Hunter DJ and Dowdeswell B (2001) Changing health care systems, *Journal of Integrated Care Pathways* 5 (2): 64–9.

Degeling P, Maxwell S, Iedema R and Hunter DJ (2004) Making clinical governance work, *British Medical Journal* 329: 679–81.

De Leeuw E, Clavier C and Breton E (2014) Health policy – why research it and how: health political science, *Health Research Policy and Systems*, 12: 55.

Department of Health (2003) *Health Check: On the State of the Public Health. Annual Report of the Chief Medical Officer.* London: Department of Health.

Department of Health (2007) *Our NHS, Our Future: NHS Next Stage Review – Interim Report.* London: Department of Health.

Department of Health (2008a) *Tackling Health Inequalities: 2007 status report on the programme for action.* London: Department of Health.

Department of Health (2008b) *Our NHS Our Future: NHS Next Stage Review – Leading Local Change.* London: Department of Health.

Department of Health and Social Security (1972) *Management Arrangements for the Reorganised National Health Service.* London: HMSO.

De Savigny D and Adam T (eds) (2009) *Systems Thinking for Health Systems Strengthening.* Geneva: Alliance for Health Policy and System Research, World Health Organisation.

Dillon A (2007) Turning theory into practice, *Health Service Journal Supplement*, Nice Guidance, 6 December.

Dixon J, Le Grand J and Smith P (2003) *Shaping the New NHS: can market forces be used for good?* London: King's Fund.

Dobbs R, Sawers C, Thompson F, Manyika J, Woetzel J, Child P, McKenna S and Spatharou A (2014) *Overcoming Obesity: an initial economic analysis*. New York, NY: McKinsey Global Institute.

Dowler E and Spencer N (eds) (2007a) *Challenging Health Inequalities: from Acheson to 'Choosing Health'*. Bristol: The Policy Press.

Dowler E and Spencer N (2007b) Challenging health inequalities: themes and issues. In: Dowler E and Spencer N (eds) *Challenging Health Inequalities: from Acheson to 'Choosing Health'*. Bristol: The Policy Press.

Draca M (2014) Institutional corruption? The revolving door in American and British politics, SMF-CAGE global perspectives series: 1.2014. www.smf.co.uk/wp-content/uploads/2014/10/Social-Market-Foundation-Insitutional-Corruption-the-revolving-door-in-American-and-British-politics.pdf.

Dunnell K (2008) Diversity and different experiences in the UK. National Statistician's Annual Article on Society. London: Office for National Statistics. www.statistics.gov.uk.

Economist Intelligence Unit (2015) *The NHS: how does it compare?* London: Economist Intelligence Unit. www.eiu.com/healthcare

Edwards B (2007) *An Independent NHS: a review of the options*. London: The Nuffield Trust.

Enthoven AC (1985) *Reflections on the Management of the National Health Service*. Occasional Papers 5. London: Nuffield Provincial Hospitals Trust.

Enthoven AC (2002) *Introducing Market Forces into Health Care: a tale of two countries*. London: The Nuffield Trust.

European Commission (2006) *Health in Europe: a strategic approach*. Discussion Document for a Health Strategy. Brussels: European Commission.

Evans RG (2005) Fellow travellers on a contested path: power, purpose and the evolution of European health care systems, *Journal of Health Politics, Policy and Law* 30 (1–2): 277–93.

Ferlie E, Pettigrew A, Ashburner L and Fitzgerald L (1996) *The New Public Management in Action*. Oxford: Oxford University Press.

Ford J and Cooke L (2000) Claims are not supported in research literature, *British Medical Journal* 321: 954.

Fotaki M (2014) *What Market-based Patient Choice can't do for the NHS: the theory of evidence of how choice works in health care.* London: Centre for Health and the Public Interest.

Fotaki M and Boyd A (2005) From plan to market: a comparison of health and old age policies in the UK and Sweden, *Public Money & Management* 25(4): 237–43.

Fotaki M, Boyd A, Smith L, McDonald R, Roland M, Sheaff R, Edwards A and Elwyn G (2005) *Patient Choice and the Organisation and Delivery of Health Services; scoping review.* A report for the NHS SDO R&D Programme. Manchester: Manchester Business School.

Francis R (2013) *Report of the Mid Staffordshire NHS Foundation Trust Public Inquiry.* HC947. London: The Stationery Office.

Freidson (1993) How dominant are the professions?, In: Hafferty FW and McKinlay JB (eds) *The Changing Medical Profession: an international perspective.* New York, NY: Oxford University Press.

Gamsu M (2015) Success lies in building stronger co-produced relationships with communities, in Local Government Association, *Devo Next: English Devolution: local solutions for a healthy nation.* London: LGA: 18-19.

Gauld R (2001) *Revolving Doors: New Zealand's health reforms.* Wellington: Institute of Policy Studies and Health Services Research Centre.

Gladwell M (2000) *The Tipping Point.* London: Abacus.

Goddard M, Hauck K, Preker A and Smith PC (2006) Priority setting in health – a political economy perspective, *Health Economics, Policy and Law* 1: 79–90.

Goldacre B (2012) *Bad Pharma: How drug companies mislead doctors and harm patients.* London: Fourth Estate.

Gorsky M (2006) Hospital governance and community involvement in Britain: evidence from before the NHS. www.historyandpolicy.org/papers/policy-paper-40.html.

Gould SJ (1990) *Wonderful Life: the Burgess Shale and the nature of history.* New York, NY: Norton.

Gray J (2003) *Al Qaeda and what it Means to be Modern.* London: Faber and Faber.

Gray J (2007) *Black Mass: apocalyptic religion and the death of utopia.* London: Allen Lane.

Greener I, Harrington BE, Hunter DJ, Mannion R and Powell M (2014) *Reforming Healthcare: what's the evidence?* Bristol: Policy Press.

Greenhalgh T, Howick J and Maskrey N (2014) Evidence based medicine: a movement in crisis?, *British Medical Journal* 348: g3725.

Greer SL and Jarman H (2007) *The Department of Health and the Civil Service: from Whitehalll to department of delivery to where?* London: The Nuffield Trust.

Greer SL, Jarman H and Azorsky A (2014) *A Reorganisation you can see from Space: The architecture of power in the new NHS.* London: Centre for Health and the Public Interest.

Griffiths R (1983) *NHS Management Inquiry Report.* London: Department of Health.

Griffiths R (1991) *Seven Years of Progress – general management in the NHS.* Audit Commission Management Lectures No 3. London: Audit Commission.

Gubb J (2007) *Just How Well Are We? A glance at trends in avoidable mortality from cancer and circulatory disease in England and Wales.* London: Civitas.

Hafferty FW and McKinlay JB (eds) (1993) *The Changing Medical Profession: an international perspective.* New York: Oxford University Press.

Haflon N, Long P, Chang DI, Hester J, Inkelas M and Rodgers A (2014) Applying a 3.0 transformation framework to guide large-scale health system reform, *Health Affairs* 33 (11): 2003-11.

Ham C (2004) *Health Policy in Britain: the politics and organisation of the NHS.* London: Palgrave Macmillan.

Ham C and Robert G (eds) (2003) *Reasonable Rationing: international experience of priority setting in health care.* Maidenhead: Open University Press.

Harrison MI (2004) *Implementing Change in Health Systems: market reforms in the UK, Sweden and The Netherlands*. London: Sage Publications.

Harrison S and Hunter DJ (1994) *Rationing Health Care*. London: Institute for Public Policy Research.

Harrison S and Pollitt C (1994) *Controlling Health Professionals: the future of work and organisation in the NHS*. Buckingham: Open University Press.

Harrison S, Hunter DJ, Marnoch G and Pollitt C (1992) *Just Managing: power and culture in the National Health Service*. Basingstoke: Macmillan.

Hastings G (2012) Why corporate power is a public health priority, *British Medical Journal* 345: e5124.

Heclo H (1975) Social politics and policy impacts. In: Holden Jr M and Dresang DL (eds) *What Government Does*. Beverly Hills: Sage.

Hood C (1991) A public management for all seasons?, *Public Administration* 69 (1): 3–19.

Hood C and Bevan G (2005) Governance by targets and terror: synecdoche, gaming and audit, *Westminster Economics Forum* 15.

Hood C and Dixon R (2015) *A Government that Worked Better and Cost Less?* Oxford: Oxford University Press.

Hopkins T and Rippon S (2015) *Head, Hands and Heart: asset-based approaches in health care*. London: The Health Foundation.

House of Commons Health Committee (2006) *Independent Sector Treatment Centres*. 4th report, session 2005–6. HC 934-I. London: The Stationery Office.

Hudson B (2015) Devo Manc: five early lessons for the NHS. *The Guardian: Healthcare Network*. www.theguardian.com/healthcare-network/2015/mar/24/devo-manc-five-early-lessons-for-the-nhs.

Hunter DJ (1980) *Coping with Uncertainty: Policy and Politics in the National Health Service*. Chichester: John Wiley & Sons Ltd.

Hunter DJ (1997) *Desperately Seeking Solutions: rationing health care*. London: Longman.

Hunter DJ (2000) Managing the NHS, *Health Care UK*. London: King's Fund: 69–76.

Hunter DJ (2005) Choosing or losing health?, *Journal of Epidemiology & Community Health* 59: 1010–12.

Hunter DJ (2006a) Efficiency. In: Marinker M (ed) *Constructive Conversations about Health: policy and values*. Oxford: Radcliffe Publishing.

Hunter DJ (2006b) From tribalism to corporatism: the continuing managerial challenge to medical dominance. In: Kelleher D, Gabe J and Williams G (eds) *Challenging Medicine*. 2nd edition. London: Routledge.

Hunter DJ (2006c) The tsunami of reform: the rise and fall of the NHS, *British Journal of Health Care Management* 12 (1): 18–23.

Hunter DJ (2007) Health improvement policy implementation in Scotland from a UK perspective. In: NHS Health Scotland *Perspectives on Health Improvement: A contribution to the consultation on the Scottish Government's action plan on health and well-being*. Edinburgh: NHS Health Scotland.

Hunter DJ (2009) Relationship between evidence and policy: a case of evidence-based policy or policy-based evidence? *Public Health* 123 (9): 583-6.

Hunter DJ (2011) Change of government: one more big bang health care reform in England's National Health Service, *International Journal of Health Services* 41 (1): 159-74.

Hunter DJ (2012) Tackling the health divide in Europe: the role of the World Health Organisation, *Journal of Health Politics, Policy and Law* 37 (5): 867-78.

Hunter DJ (2013) *To Market! To Market!* London: Centre for Health and the Public Interest.

Hunter DJ (2015a) Health policy and management: in praise of political science, *International Journal of Health Policy and Management* 4:1-4.

Hunter DJ (2015b) Role of politics in understanding complex, messy health systems: an essay, *British Medical Journal* 350: h1214.

Hunter DJ and Marks L (2005) *Managing for Health: what incentives exist for NHS managers to focus on wider health issues?* London: King's Fund.

Hunter DJ and Williams G (2012) NHS 'reform' in England: where is the public interest? *British Medical Journal* 344: e2014. Doi: 10.1136/bmj.e2014

Hunter DJ and Williamson P (1991) Comparisons and contrasts between Scotland and England, *Health Services Management* 87 (4): 166-70.

Hunter DJ and Wistow G (1987) *Community Care in Britain: variations on a theme.* London: King Edward's Hospital Fund for London.

Hunter DJ, Erskine J, Hicks C, McGovern T, Small A, Lugsden E, Whitty P, Steen IH and Eccles M (2014) A mixed-methods evaluation of transformational change in NHS North East, *Health Services and Delivery Research* 2 (47).

Hunter DJ, Erskine J, Small A, McGovern T, Hicks C, Whitty P and Lugsden E (2015) Doing transformational change in the English NHS in the context of 'big bang' redisorganisation: findings from the North East Transformational System, *Journal of Health Organisation and Management* 29(1): 10-24.

Hunter DJ, Schrecker T and Alderslade R (2015) Guest editors special issue, Governance for health in a changing world, *Public Health* 129 (7): 831-2.

Hunter DJ, Marks L and Smith KE (2010) *The Public Health System in England.* Bristol: The Policy Press.

Hunter DJ, Shishkin S and Taroni F (2005) Steering the purchaser: stewardship and government. In: Figueras J, Robinson R and Jakubowski E (eds) *Purchasing to Improve Health Systems Performance.* Maidenhead: Open University Press.

Institute of Medicine (2003) *The Future of the Public's Health in the 21st Century.* Washington, DC: The National Academies Press.

Jakab Z and Alderslade R (2015) Health 2020 – achieving health and development in today's Europe, *Global Policy* 6 (2): 166-171. DOI: 10.1111/1758-5899.12166

James O (2007) *Affluenza.* London: Vermilion.

James O and Manning N (1996) Public management reform – a global perspective, *Politics* 16(3): 143–9.

Johnson A (2007) *The Healthy Society,* speech by Alan Johnson, Secretary of State for Health, 12 September. London: Department of Health, http://webarchive.nationalarchives. gov.uk/201330107105354/http://www.dh.gov.uk/en/ MediaCentre/Speeches/DH_078397

Jones O (2015) *The Establishment and How They Get Away with it.* London: Penguin.

Judt T (2010) *Ill Fares the Land: a treatise on our present discontents.* London: Penguin.

Jupp B (2015) *Reconsidering Accountability in an Age of Integrated Care. Viewpoint.* London: The Nuffield Trust.

Kawachi I (2007) Individual versus collective responsibility for health (or why some societies make you sick). Presentation to UKPHA Annual Public Health Forum 2007, Edinburgh. www. ukpha.org.uk.

Kawachi I, Kennedy BP, Lochner K and Prothrow-Stith D (1997) Social capital, income and inequality, *American Journal of Public Health* 87: 1491–8.

Kelly MP (2007) Evidence-based public health. In: Griffiths S and Hunter DJ (eds) *New Perspectives in Public Health.* 2nd edition. Oxford: Radcliffe Publishing.

Kerr D (2005) *Building a Health Service Fit for the Future.* Edinburgh: The Scottish Government.

Kerr D and Feeley D (2007) Collectivism and collaboration in NHS Scotland. In: Greer SL and Rowland D (eds) *Devolving Policy, Diverging Values? The values of the United Kingdom's health services.* London: The Nuffield Trust.

Kettl DF (1993) *Sharing Power: public governance and private markets.* Washington, DC: The Brookings Institution.

Kickbusch I (2004) The Leavell Lecture – The end of public health as we know it: constructing global health in the 21st century, *Public Health,* 118 (7): 463–9.

Kickbusch I (2007) Health governance: the health society. In: McQueen D, Kickbusch I et al *Health Modernity: the role of theory in health promotion*. New York: Springer.

King A and Crewe I (2014) *The Blunders of our Governments*. London: Oneworld.

Kingdon J (1986) *Agendas, alternatives and public policies*, New York, NY: Little Brown.

Klein R (1971) Accountability in the NHS, *Political Quarterly* 42: 363-75.

Klein R (1983) Comment on chapter 7. In: Young K (ed) *National Interests and Local Government*. Joint Studies in Public Policy 7. London: Heinemann.

Klein R (1995) Big bang health care reform – does it work? The case of Britain's National Health Service reform, *Milbank Quarterly* 73(3): 299-337.

Klein R (2006) *The New Politics of the NHS*. 5th edition. Oxford: Radcliffe Publishing.

Klein R (2007) Editorial: rationing in the NHS, *British Medical Journal* 334: 1068-9.

Klein R and Marmor TR (2006) Reflections on policy analysis: putting it together again. In: Moran M, Rein M and Goodin RE (eds) *The Oxford Handbook of Public Policy*. Oxford: Oxford University Press.

Kraanen F and Meerkerk C (2006) *Taking Care of Tomorrow*. Amsterdam: Ministry of Health, Welfare and Sport.

Lancet, The (1995) Editorial: market futures, fantasies and fallacies, *The Lancet* 346, 8 July: 63.

Lang T and Rayner G (2012) Ecological public health: the 21st century's big idea. An essay, *British Medical Journal* 345: e5466.

Laffin M (2007) Comparative British central–local relations: regional centralism, governance and intergovernmental relations, *Public Policy and Administration* 22 (1): 74–91.

Lasswell HD (1936) *Politics: who gets what, when, how*. New York, NY: Whittlesey House.

Laughlin R (1991) Environmental disturbances and organisational transitions and transformations: some alternative models, *Organisation Studies* 12(2): 209–32.

Lawson N (2007) *Machines, Markets and Morals: the new politics of a democratic NHS.* London: Compass.

Layard R (2005) *Happiness: lessons from a new science.* London: Penguin Press.

Layard R (2006) *Happiness: lessons from a new science.* 2nd edition. London: Penguin.

Le Grand (2003) *Motivation, Agency and Public Policy: of knights and knaves, pawns and queens.* Oxford: Oxford University Press.

Le Grand J (2007) *The Other Invisible Hand.* New Jersey and London: Princeton University Press.

Leadbeater C (2004) *Personalisation through Participation: a new script for public services.* London: Demos.

Lenaghan J (1996) *Rationing and Rights in Health Care.* London: Institute for Public Policy Research.

Leppo K (1998) Introduction. In: Koivisalu M and Ollilia E (eds) *Making a Healthy World.* London: Zed Books.

Letwin O and Redwood J (1988) *Britain's Biggest Enterprise: ideas for radical reform of the NHS.* London: Centre for Policy Studies.

Leys C and Player S (2011) *The Plot against the NHS.* London: Merlin Press.

Light DW and Hughes D (2002) Introduction: a sociological perspective on rationing: power, rhetoric and situated practices. In: Hughes D and Light D (eds) *Rationing: constructed realities and professional practices.* Oxford: Blackwell.

Lipsky M (1980) *Street Level Bureaucracy.* New York, NY: Sage Foundation.

Local Government Association (2015) *Devo Next. English Devolution: local solutions for a healthy nation.* London: Local Government Association.

Longley M, Riley N, Davies P, Hernandez-Quevedo C (2012) United Kingdom (Wales) Health system review, *Health Systems in Transition* 14 (11): 1-84.

Loughlin M (1996) The language of quality. *Journal of Evaluation in Clinical Practice* 2(2): 87-95.

Maarse H (ed) (2004) *Privatisation in European Health Care. A comparative analysis in eight countries.* Maarssen: Elsevier.

Mackenbach JP (2005) *Health Inequalities: Europe in profile.* London: UK Presidency of the EU.

Mackenbach JP (2010) Has the English strategy to reduce health inequalities failed? *Social Science & Medicine* 71: 1249-53.

Mackenzie WJM (1979) *Power and Responsibility in Health Care.* London: Oxford University Press for Nuffield Provincial Hospitals Trust.

Madelin R (2006) UK Health challenges: can the EU make a difference?, *Clinical Medicine* 6(5): 493–6.

Marks L and Hunter DJ (2005) *Practice Based Commissioning: Policy into Practice.* Bath: Medical Management Services.

Marks L and Hunter DJ (2007) *Social Enterprises and the NHS: changing patterns of ownership and accountability.* London: UNISON.

Marmor T (2004) *Fads in Medical Care Management and Policy.* Rock Carling Fellowship. London: Nuffield Trust and The Stationery Office.

Marmor TR, Mashaw JL and Harvey PL (eds) (1990) *America's Misunderstood Welfare State: persisting myths, enduring realities.* New York, NY: Basic Books.

Marmor T and Klein R (2012) *Politics, Health and Health Care: selected essays.* New Haven, CT and London:Yale University Press.

Marmot M (2010) *Fair Society, Healthy Lives.* The Marmot Review. Strategic Review of Health Inequalities in England post-2010. London: University College London.

McDonald R (2002) *Using Health Economics in Health Services: rationing rationally?* Buckingham: Open University Press.

McKee M, Hurst L, Aldridge RW, Rane R, Mindell JS, Wolfe I and Holland WW (2011) Public health in England: an option for the way forward? *The Lancet* 378(9790): 536-9.

McMichael T and Beaglehole R (2004) The global context for public health. In: Beaglehole R (ed) *Global Public Health: a new era*. Oxford: Oxford University Press.

Mechanic D (1995) Dilemmas in rationing health care services: the case for implicit rationing, *British Medical Journal* 310: 1655–9.

Meek J (2014) *Private Island: Why Britain now belongs to someone else*. London: Verso.

Milburn A (2002) Tackling health inequalities: improving public health. Lecture to the Faculty of Public Health Medicine. London: Department of Health.

Miller H (1973) *Medicine and Society*. Oxford: Oxford University Press.

Mohan J (2002) *Planning, Markets and Hospitals*. London: Routledge.

Mohan J (2003) The past and future of the NHS: New Labour and foundation hospitals. www.historyandpolicy.org/papers/policy-paper-14.html.

Mooney G (2012) Neoliberalism is bad for our health, *International Journal of Health Services* 42 (3): 383-401.

Morgan A and Ziglio E (2007) Revitalising the evidence base for public health: an assets model, *Promotion & Education* Supplement 2: 17–22.

National Audit Office (2010) *Department of Health. Tackling inequalities in life expectancy in areas with the worst health and deprivation*. HC 186 Session 2010-11. London: The Stationery Office.

National Consumer Council (1998) *Consumer Concerns 1998 – a consumer view of health services*. The report of an RSL survey. London: National Consumer Council.

www.nice.org.uk/news/article/wider-use-of-statins-could-cut-deaths-from-heart-disease.

Needham C (2008a) *The Reform of Public Services under New Labour: narratives of consumerism*. Basingstoke: Palgrave.

Needham C (2008b) Realising the potential of co-production: negotiating improvements in public services, *Social Policy & Society* 7 (2): 221–31.

New Economics Foundation (2006) *Behavioural Economics: seven principles for policy-makers.* London: New Economics Foundation.

NHS England (2014) *The National Health Service Five Year Forward View.* London: NHS England.

NICE (National Institute for Health and Care Excellence) (2014) Wider use of statins could cut deaths from heart disease, 18 July. www.nice.org.uk.

Nolte E and McKee M (2004) *Does Healthcare Save Lives? Avoidable mortality revisited.* London: The Nuffield Trust.

Nuffield Council on Bioethics (2007) *Public Health: ethical issues.* London: Nuffield Council on Bioethics.

O'Neill C, McGregor P and Merkur S (2012) United Kingdom (Northern Ireland) Health system review, *Health Systems in Transition* 14 (10): 1-91.

Office for National Statistics (2008) *Social Trends 38.* London: ONS. www.statistics.gov.uk/socialtrends38.

Oliver A and Mossialos E (2005) European health systems reforms: looking backward to see forward?, *Journal of Health Politics, Policy and Law*, 30 (1–2): 7–28.

Osborne D and Gaebler T (1993) *Reinventing government: How the entrepreneurial spirit is transforming the public sector.* New York, NY: Plume.

Osborne SP and McLaughlin K (2002) The new public management in context. In: McLaughlin K, Osborne SP and Ferlie E (eds) *New Public Management: current trends and future prospects.* London: Routledge.

Ottersen OP, Frenk J and Horton R (2014) The Lancet-University of Oslo Commission on Global Governance for Health, *The Lancet* 378 (9803): 1612-3.

Owen D (2014) *The Health of the Nation: NHS in peril.* York: Methuen.

Paine D (2015) Health secretary could overturn devolved decisions, *Health Service Journal,* 26 June.

Paton C (2006) *New Labour's State of Health: political economy, public policy and the NHS.* Aldershot: Ashgate.

Paton C (2014) Garbage-can policy-making meets neo-liberal ideology: twenty five years of redundant reform of the English National Health Service, *Social Policy & Administration* 48 (3): 319-42.

Pfeffer J (1992) *Managing with Power: politics and influence in organisations*. Boston, MA: Harvard Business School Press.

Plsek P and Greenhalgh T (2001) The challenge of complexity in health care, *British Medical Journal* 323: 625-8.

Pollitt C (1993) *Managerialism and the Public Services*. 2nd edition. Oxford: Blackwell.

Pollock AM (2005) *NHS plc: the privatisation of our health care*. London: Verso.

Pollock AM (2015) *The End of the NHS*. London: Verso.

Pollock A, Macfarlane A, Kirkwood G, Majeed FA, Greener I, Morelli C et al (2011) No evidence that patient choice saves lives, *The Lancet*, 378: 2057-60.

Popay J, Whitehead M and Hunter DJ (2010) Injustice is killing people on a large scale – but what is to be done about it?, *Journal of Public Health* 32 (2): 150-6.

Porter M and Teisberg E (2006) *Redefining Health Care: creating value-based competition on results*. Boston, MA: Harvard Business School Press.

Powell I (2005) Moving forward or backwards in the health system; new and old stories. Address to New Zealand Society of Hospital and Community Dentistry, 30 July, Auckland, New Zealand (unpublished).

Power M (1997) *The Audit Society: rituals of verification*. Oxford: Clarendon Press.

Propper C, Sutton M, Whitnall C, Windmeijer F (2008) Did 'targets and terror' reduce waiting times in England for hospital care? *B E Journal of Economic Analysis and Policy* 8 (2).

Ranade W (1998) *Markets and Health Care: a comparaive analysis*. London: Longman.

Rawlins MD (2015) National Institute for Clinical Excellence: NICE works, *Journal of the Royal Society of Medicine* 108 (6): 211-19.

Rhodes RAW (1996) The new governance: governing without government, *Political Studies* 44: 652–667.

Rid A, Littlejohns P, Wilson J, Rumbold B, Kieslich K and Weale A (2015) The importance of being NICE, *Journal of the Royal Society of Medicine Online First*, 2 October: 1–5.

Rummery K and McAngus C (2015) The future of social policy in Scotland: will further devolved powers lead to better social policies for disabled people? *The Political Quarterly* 86 (2): 234-39.

Saltman RB and von Otter C (1992) *Planned Markets and Public Competition: strategic reform in Northern European health systems.* Buckingham: Open University Press.

Saltman RB and Bergman S-E (2005) Renovating the commons: Swedish health care reforms in perspective, *Journal of Health Politics, Policy and Law* 30(1–2): 253–75.

Sandel MJ (2013) *What money Can't Buy: the moral limits of markets.* London: Penguin.

Savage W (2006) Foreword. In: Nunns A *The 'Patchwork Privatisation' of our Health Service: a users' guide.* London: Keep Our NHS Public. www.keepournhspublic.com.

Schrecker T and Bambra C (2015) *How Politics Makes Us Sick: Neoliberal epidemics.* Basingstoke: Palgrave Macmillan.

Schon D (1973) *Beyond the Stable State.* Harmondsworth: Penguin.

Secretary of State for Health (2004) *Choosing Health: making healthier choices easier.* Cm 6374. London: The Stationery Office.

Secretary of State for Health (2010a) *Healthy Lives, Healthy People: our strategy for public health in England.* Cm 7985. London: The Stationery Office.

Secretary of State for Health (2010b) *Equity and Excellence: liberating the NHS.* Cm 7881. London: The Stationery Office.

Seddon J (2003) *Freedom from Command and Control: a better way to make the work work.* Buckingham: Vanguard Education.

Sen A (2015) The economic consequences of austerity, *New Statesman* 5-11 June: 29-33.

Sennett R (1999) *The Corrosion of Character: the personal consequences of work in the new capitalism.* London: Norton & Co.

Sennett R (2006) *The Culture of the New Capitalism.* New Haven: Yale University Press.

Sennett R (2008) *The Craftsman.* London: Allen Lane.

Shipman Inquiry (2004) *Safeguarding Patients: lessons from the past – proposals for the future.* 5th report. Cm 6394 (Chair: Dame Janet Smith). London: The Stationery Office.

Simon HA (1957) *Administrative Behaviour.* New York, NY: Free Press.

Smith I (2006) *Building a World-class NHS,* London: Reform.

Smith K, Hunter DJ, Blackman T et al (2008) Divergence or convergence? Health inequalities and policy in a devolved Britain, *Critical Social Policy* (in press).

Smith J, Porter A, Shaw S, Rosen R, Blunt I and Mays N (2013) *Commissioning High-Quality Care for People with Long-Term Conditions.* London: Nuffield Trust.

Smith P (2003) The case against the internal market. In: Dixon J, Le Grand J and Smith P *Shaping the New NHS: can market forces be used for good?* London: King's Fund.

Stahl T, Wismar M, Ollila E, Lahtinen E and Leppo K (eds) (2006) *Health in All Policies: prospects and potentials.* Helsinki: Finnish Ministry of Social Affairs and Health and European Observatory on Health Systems and Policies.

Stevens R (2007) *The Public-Private Health Care State: essays on the history of American health care policy.* New Brunswick, NJ and London: Transaction Publishers.

Steel D and Cylus J (2012) United Kingdom (Scotland): health system review, *Health Systems in Transition* 14 (9): 1-150.

Stevens S (2004) Reform strategies for the English NHS, *Health Affairs* 23 (3): 37–44.

Stevens S (2010) NHS reform is a risk worth taking. The new plans move toward fulfilling Blair's vision, *Financial Times* 15 July www.ft.com/cms/s/0/2932b84e-904a-11df-ad26-00144feab49a.html#axzz3ep2UNM37.

Stewart J (1998) Advance or retreat: from the traditions of public administration to the new public management and beyond, *Public Policy and Administration* 13 (4): 12–27.

Strauss A, Schatzman L, Bucher R, Ehrlich D and Sabshin M (1964) *Psychiatric Ideologies and Institutions.* New York, NY: Free Press.

Street A (2015) Tax-based financing of the NHS is better than the alternatives, *The Conversation* 23 April.

Stuckler D and Basu S (2013) *The Body Economic: why austerity kills.* London: Allen Lane.

Taylor-Gooby P and Stoker G (2011) The coalition programme: a new vision for Britain or politics as usual? *The Political Quarterly* 82 (1): 4-15.

Thaler RH and Sunstein CR (2008) *Nudge: improving decisions about health, wealth and happiness,* New Haven: Yale University Press.

Tedstone A, Targett V, Allen R and staff at PHE (2015) *Sugar reduction: The evidence for action,* London: Public Health England.

Timmins N (1995) *The Five Giants: a biography of the welfare state.* London: HarperCollins.

Timmins N (2012) *Never Again? The story of the Health and Social Care Act 2012.* London: King's Fund.

Timmins N (2013) *The Four UK Health Systems: learning from each other.* London: King's Fund.

Timmins N (2015) *Practice of System Leadership: being comfortable with chaos.* London: King's Fund.

Torgerson DJ and Gosden T (2000) Priority setting in health care: should we ask the tax payer? *British Medical Journal* 320: 1679.

Travis P, Egger D, Davies P and Mechbal A (2002) *Towards Better Stewardship: concepts and critical issues.* Geneva: World Health Organisation.

Tudor Hart J (1971) The inverse care law, *The Lancet* 1: 404–12.

Tudor Hart J (1994) *Feasible Socialism: the NHS past, present and future.* London: Socialist Health Association.

Ubel PA (2001) Physicians, thou shalt ration: the necessary role of bedside rationing in controlling healthcare costs, *Healthcare Papers* 2 (2): 10–21.

Wanless D (2002) *Securing Our Future Health: taking a long-term view.* London: HM Treasury.

Wanless D (2004) *Securing Good Health for the Whole Population.* Final report. London: HM Treasury.

Wanless D, Appleby J, Harrison A and Patel D (2007) *Our future Health Secured? A review of NHS funding and performance.* London: King's Fund.

Webster C (2002) *The National Health Service: a political history.* New edition. Oxford: Oxford University Press.

West D (2014) Exclusive: Patient choice is not key to improving performance, says Hunt. *Health Service Journal* 26 November, http://m.hsj.co.uk/5077051.article

Westert GP and Verkleij H (eds) (2006) *Dutch Health Care Performance Report 2006.* Bilthoven: National Institute for Public Health and the Environment.

White J (2007) Markets and medical care: the United States, 1993–2005, *Milbank Quarterly* 85 (3): 1–29.

Whitehead M (2014) *Due North: the report of the inquiry on health equity for the North.* Liverpool: University of Liverpool and Centre for Local Economic Strategies.

Whitley R (1988) The management sciences and managerial skills, *Organisation Studies* 9 (1): 47–68.

WHO (World Health Organisation) (2000) *The World Health Report 2000 – health systems: improving performance.* Geneva: WHO.

WHO (2005) *Strengthened Health Systems Save More Lives. An insight into WHO's European health systems' strategy.* Copenhagen: WHO.

WHO (2012a) *Health 2020: a European policy framework and strategy for the 21st century.* Copenhagen: WHO Regional Office for Europe.

WHO (2012b) *European Action Plan for Strengthening Public Health Capacities and Services.* Copenhagen: WHO Regional Office for Europe.

WHO (2015) *Health in All Policies (HiAP): Training Manual.* Geneva: WHO.

Wilks S (2013) *The Political Power of the Business Corporation*, Cheltenham: Edward Elgar.

Wilkinson RG (2005) *The Impact of Inequality: how to make sick societies healthier.* London: Routledge.

Wilkinson R and Pickett K (2009) *The Spirit Level: why more equal societies almost always do better.* London: Allen Lane.

Williams I, Robinson S and Dickinson H (2012) *Rationing in Health Care: the theory and practice of priority-setting,* Bristol: The Policy Press.

Williams J and Rossiter A (2004) *Choice: the evidence. The operation of choice systems in practice: national and international evidence.* London: Social Market Foundation.

Wise M and Nutbeam D (2007) Enabling health systems transformation: what progress has been made in re-orienting health services?, *Promotion & Education* Supplement 2: 23–7.

Woolhandler S and Himmelstein DU (2007) Competition in a publicly funded healthcare system, *British Medical Journal* 335: 1126–9.

World Bank (1993) *World Development Report 1993: investing in health.* Oxford: Oxford University Press.

Index